WE DON'T BUY SICKNESS, IT JUST COMES

We Don't Buy Sickness, It Just Comes

Health, Illness and Health Care in the Lives of Black People in London

JENNY DONOVAN
*The Medical School,
University of Birmingham*

Gower

Published by

Gower Publishing Company Limited,
Gower House,
Croft Road,
Aldershot,
Hants GU11 3HR
England.

Gower Publishing Company,
Old Post Road,
Brookfield,
Vermont 05036
USA.

Reprinted 1993

British Library Cataloguing in Publication Data

Donovan, Jenny
We don't buy sickness, it just comes : health, illness and health care in the lives of black people in London.
1. Minorities——Health and hygiene——England——London
I. Title
305.8'009421 RA408.M/

Library of Congress Cataloging-in-Publication Data

Donovan, Jenny, 1960-
We don't buy sickness, it just comes.

Bibliography: p.
1. Blacks--Health and hygiene--England--London.
2. Blacks--Medical care--England--London. 3. South Asians--Health and hygiene--England--London. 4. South Asians--Medical care--England--London. I. Title.
[DNLM: 1. Blacks. 2. Ethnic Groups--London. 3. Health Services--London. 4. Health Surveys--London.
5. Morbidity--London. WA 900 FA1 D6w]
RA488.L8D65 1986 362.1'08996'0421 86-7672

ISBN: 0 566 05201 6

Printed in Great Britain

Contents

Tables

Figures

Abstract

The thesis is concerned with the perceptions and experiences of health, illness and health care of thirty people of Afro-Caribbean and Asian descent living in London. It opens with an overview of the history of black immigration, settlement and race relations in post world-war-two Britain. The importance of "culture" is assessed, particularly its effects on health and its use in place of, or alongside, "race." The introductory chapters are concluded by a review of the research undertaken specifically on illnesses and diseases suffered by members of ethnic groups, and the reasons for the concentration on some groups and conditions at the expense of others are considered.

The main body of the thesis concerns the empirical work with thirty people of Afro-Caribbean and Asian descent. Attention is given to the methodology of the study, and the relevance of interpretative sociology and ethnography are assessed. The concentration on a relatively small number of cases and the use of in-depth interviewing techniques are explained. The empirical work itself is reported in detail in two chapters, thus allowing the reader to see from where the author's interpretations arise.

The thesis is concluded by a chapter whose aim is to evaluate the methodology and integrate the introductory chapters with the ethnography. Here, the links between the subjects' perceptions and experiences, the history of immigration, the concept of culture, the importance of racism and other contemporary social, political and economic forces are analysed, and the health and lives of the subjects are placed in their social context.

Preface

It is the aim of this thesis to examine and understand the perceptions and experiences of health, ill-health and the health services of two groups of black people living in London. The study is set in the context of the history of immigration and race relations in Britain since the second world war. Relevant topics whose importance is to be investigated include racism and culture. The methodology of the study is located within a recent move in human geography towards the exploration of more qualitative methods, drawing particularly on ethnography, interpretative sociology and the case-study approach (see, for example, Mitchell, 1983; Jackson and Smith, 1984). The bulk of the thesis is taken up by an ethnography of empirical work reproduced in detail so that the reader is able to see from where interpretations arise.

Chapter one concerns the broad context of the study. Overall, there is a confusion of terms used in research on black people. The word "immigrant" is used, for example, to denote "black", when in fact this is increasingly inappropriate as more blacks are born in Britain. Immigrants include a wide range of ethnicities and nationalities, by no means all of whom are of so-called New Commonwealth origin. The word "immigrant" is also pejorative in tone and indicative of an outsider. Words and phrases such as "ethnic minority", "non-white", "Asian" and so on are often used indiscriminately, and without adequate definition. In this thesis, the term "Asian" is used to refer to people of Indian, Pakistani or Bangladeshi descent; and "Afro-Caribbean" to refer to people of African or West Indian descent. "Minority", "ethnic" or "ethnic minority" group are also used to describe any group of people who share a common heritage and are not part of the majority society. "Black" is also used. This is a political term, emphasising solidarity and unity between minority groups discriminated against because of the colour of their skin (ILEA, 1983). In this thesis, "black" refers to people of Asian and Afro-Caribbean descent who share the common experience of racial discrimination because of the colour of their skin.

Before moving on to establish the context within which the study is set, I would like to thank all those who have helped me to get this far. I would particularly like to thank Dr John Eyles of QMC for his encouragement and enthusiasm for the project; and Professor David Smith, also of QMC, for his help and critical comments. I am also indebted to Prince Owusu-Sekyere, Surriya, Rita, Peter McCarthy and Humphrey Southall, who have all proved crucial in a variety of ways and at different times. I must also thank Sarah Curtis, Maggie Pearson and Caroline Sikorski for their help. Thanks are also due to John Youd at QMC who drew up the figures. The project was funded for three years by the SSRC/ESRC.

It remains for me to add my final and greatest thanks to the thirty people who are this project. Without them, I would know nothing.

PART I
THE THEORETICAL BACKGROUND

These theories of racial superiority and inferiority which developed in part to justify imperial exploitation, still have some influence today. "Race" is still used as a pseudo-biological category (van den Burghe, 1978), applied according to visible, rather than any true biological differences. Out of this conception of race have grown the concepts of "racialism" and "racism", both of which have variable definitions, depending on the political leaning of the definer and on the historical context.

Some definitions of racism tend to refer to the issue of the hierarchy of the races: (Racism is) "The doctrine that a man's [sic] behaviour is determined by stable and inheritable characteristics deriving from separate racial stocks having distinctive attributes and usually considered to stand to one another in relations of superiority and inferiority" (Banton, 1967, 81); (Racism is the) "Dogma that one group is condemned by nature to congenital inferiority and another to superiority" (Clarke, Ley and Peach, 1984, 14). Phizacklea and Miles (1980) also ascribe to the view that racism is a set of negative beliefs held by a group which identifies another on the grounds of biological or inheritable characteristics. These three views see racism as being derived directly from the ideas of the Social Darwinists.

Other writers define racism in terms of power. Wilson, (1973), for example, sees racism as the ideology of racial domination or exploitation which incorporates beliefs in a particular race's inferiority and uses such beliefs to justify or prescribe unequal treatment for that group. Rex (1983) and Lewis (1973) see racism as a theory developed by one group to justify its privileged position over another. Bourne and Sivanandan (1980) declare that racism is defined simply by the power of whites over blacks.

For some writers, racism is just one expression of the capitalist mode of production (Cox, 1948; Cooper, 1983), but this conception ignores the existence of racism in non- or pre-capitalist societies such as the USSR, Cuba and pre-capitalist Europe. Racism may, alternatively, be the theory that human activities are determined by race (Pillary, 1984). The Centre for Contemporary Cultural Studies has produced a package of similar definitions of racism: Hall suggests that racism is historically specific (1978), and that it is built into the fabric of institutions such as housing and employment; Solomos et al (1982), like Cox and Cooper above, claim that racism is part of capitalist development; and Lawrence (1982) sees racism as a theory which has grown out of the history of the Empire, colonisation and immigration, and which is an organic component of the contemporary crisis. Barker (1981) sees racism as any theory which supports the idea that it is "natural" to feel hostility towards certain groups.

No single author seems, then, to have achieved a satisfactory definition of racism. Van den Burghe (1978) feels that no single definition is achievable, because racism means different things to writers with different approaches. Similarly, Banton (1977), suggests that the word "racism" carries with it too many ideas, and so has lost its usefulness. In this thesis, racism is considered to include a constellation of ideas: racism is a theory which has grown out of xenophobia, uneven power-relations and colonialism, and which encourages or allows the unequal treatment of some people on the basis that they are inferior or different. Racist theories are historically specific, moulding themselves to contemporary beliefs and demands. Their existence may be inferred from literary writing, vernacular language, historical documentation and contemporary press and social surveys.

"Racialism" is now a word used sparingly. It refers, typically, to the practice of the theory of racism (Rex, 1983; Contemp. Issues in Geog. and Educ., 1983). Bourne and Sivanandan (1980), however, define racialism as the cultural intolerance underlying racial discrimination. Things cultural are defined by the majority of writers, however, as the concerns of ethnicity (van den Burghe, 1978; Watson, 1977; Lawrence, 1982b; Cohen, 1974).

Racism has had an important role in maintaining and justifying European domination and exploitation over the third world and over black workers in the developed world (Baran and Sweezy, 1966). The Social Darwinists justified imperialism by developing theories which claimed to prove the superiority of the white race over the black. Black cultures were labelled "primitive", and Africans in particular were seen as uncivilised and childlike (Lawrence, 1982a). Thus the use of slaves was justified, because it was the "inevitable" outcome of their inferiority to whites; and colonial rule accepted because of the inability of the "natives" to rule themselves as well as the English could. At home, the use of slaves or black servants re-inforced these views, and the reading of "sambo" stories and teaching of the imperialist version of history helped to instill racist images into children's minds. The English language can also be seen to have incorporated racist ideas with the association of dirtiness, death, darkness and wickedness with "black", compared with the association of purity, perfection, cleanness, light and goodness with "white" (Jordan, 1982). Similarly, words such as coon, wog, yid and Paki have been, and still are, used to denote specific racial or ethnic groups. To ignore the importance of these and other images in today's racism would be to ignore the history and bases for discrimination. The crucial importance of these images lies, however, in their manipulation by contemporary political figures (see chapter two).

IMMIGRATION AND WHITE REACTION

Immigration is not a modern phenomenon in Britain : it has been happening for many centuries. Black people have been seen in this country since the times of Elizabeth I (Fryer, 1984), and were brought in larger numbers in the seventeenth century as slaves. In the 1770s and 1780s, some 10,000 slaves are thought to have been in Britain (Shyllon, 1977). Before 1905, there were no official restrictions on who could enter Britain and settle here, and there were well-established groups of long-term resident Jews, blacks and Irish.

Large scale Irish immigration occurred mainly between 1800 and 1861, with their coming to find work and to escape from poverty and famine in Ireland (Jones, 1977). The majority were unskilled, and they settled chiefly at the ends of steamship routes, in Liverpool and London particularly. An estimate of the number of Irish people living in Britain in 1841 was about 1.8 per cent of the population of England and Wales. By 1861, this had risen to 3 per cent. According to the Appendix to the Poor Law Report of the time, Ireland was generally seen by the British to be a backward country, and there were complaints that the Irish immigrants were dirty, had low levels of health, and that they threatened to reduce wage levels and take all the jobs (Jones, 1977).

The next wave of immigrants were Eastern European Jews who arrived from 1870 to 1911. They came from Russia, Poland and Rumania, often escaping from persecution and pogroms. Some 280,000 Jews had arrived in Britain by 1911, and 60% of these settled in the East End of London, particularly in Stepney (Jones, ibid). They were linguistically and culturally more foreign and "strange" than the Irish, and there were concerns expressed about their levels of hygiene and low standards of living, as well as the threats they were thought to pose to public health, morals, and law and order. In cartoons and the popular media, Jews were seen to be scheming, mean and crafty. The government responded to popular complaints about the numbers of "alien" Jews by introducing the Aliens Restrictions Acts of 1905 and 1914 (Rees, 1982). These Acts sought to prevent "undesirable and destitute aliens" from settling in Britain, and meant that only Jews who could prove that they were "bona fide" refugees from religious persecution were allowed to settle (Jones, 1977). These Acts set the precedent for dealing with immigrants by legislating against them.

It was not until after World War II that large-scale immigration to Britain occurred again. Immediately after the end of the war, some Polish immigrants applied to settle in Britain rather than returning to Poland, and they were allowed to do so. Plans for the rebuilding of industry after the war led to increased demand for labour. The boom of the 1950s added to the pressure for labour and accentuated the shortage of indigenous workers. Coincidentally, owing to the nature of colonial and neo-colonial development, there were vast reserves of un- and under-employed workers in the Caribbean and Indian sub-continent.

The attraction of job opportunities in the "mother country" caused people from the West Indies to migrate to Britain from the late 1940s onwards (Peach, 1968). Conditions in the West Indies were an important factor in allowing emigration, especially the high levels of unemployment and population pressure, but the perceived job opportunities in Britain were the principal causal factor. There were very close correlations between seasonal cycles of employment in the UK and immigration rates from the West Indies (Peach, ibid; Philpott, 1973; Foner, 1979). Perceived opportunities were not the only "pull", however, as organisations such as London Transport, British Rail and other smaller concerns recruited workers directly from Barbados and Jamaica. These people were required to do jobs that had not been filled by white workers, either because there were not enough of them, or because the jobs were unattractive owing to their low pay and poor conditions.

The period between the end of World War II and 1962 has been termed a "laissez-faire" immigration period (Sivanandan, 1982), because it was then part of the constitution that there should be no restrictions on residents of empire territories who wanted to work or settle in Britain. Under the terms of Independence too, all inhabitants of British colonies were entitled to full British passports and thus the same rights of entry and abode in the UK as British residents. This became particularly important after the passing in the US of the McCurren-Walter Act of 1952 which restricted the numbers of immigrants from the West Indies to the USA, and made the UK the target for most migrants.

The amount of immigration from India and Pakistan was small during this period because it was largely controlled by the governments of India and Pakistan and was limited mainly to professionals or ex-forces personnel. The majority of immigrants to Britain between 1948 and 1960 were from the Caribbean. By 1960, there were 161,450 people of West Indian birth in Britain compared with only 33,070 from India and 17,120 from Pakistan (Jones, 1977).

After 1960, the pattern began to change. The 1959 general election campaign produced a proposal for a Commonwealth Immigrants Bill which was later introduced by the Conservative government. The aim of the Bill was to limit and control immigration from the New Commonwealth and Pakistan (ie the black ex-colonies) through a system of work vouchers which people would have to apply for and whose numbers could be monitored and controlled. Many of the immigrants already settled in Britain urged their friends and relatives to come over, fearing that if they did not do so soon, they would not be able to come at all (Hiro, 1973). Consequently, far from limiting immigration in the short term, the Bill caused a huge increase in numbers, with 49,000 arriving from the West Indies in 1960 compared with 16,400 in 1959; and 48,000 arriving from India and Pakistan in 1961 compared with 7,500 in 1960. By 1961, there were 522,933 people of New Commonwealth and Pakistan origin in Britain; and the impending Act had caused many of those who had originally planned to return to their countries of origin to decide to settle permanently in the UK and to bring over their families.

The Commonwealth Immigrants Act was passed in 1962. The Act restricted primary immigration by establishing three categories of employment vouchers. Category "A" vouchers were issued only to people with specific jobs to go to; "B" vouchers to people with "specific marketable skills"; and "C" vouchers to unskilled workers without specific prospects of employment. Category "C" vouchers were abolished in 1965, and between 1962 and 1965, only 10% of these had gone to people in the Caribbean, the rest going to Indians and Pakistanis, thus reversing the earlier pattern of immigration. In 1963, for example, there were only 7,928 arrivals from the West Indies, compared with 17,498 from India and 16,336 from Pakistan (Jones, 1977).

The passing of the Commonwealth Immigrants Act meant that black immigration was restricted. The Act aimed to limit immigration only from the "new" black Commonwealth - the West Indies, India and Pakistan - not the "old" Commonwealth of Canada, New Zealand and Australia (Sivanandan, 1983). After the passing of the Act, black immigration became an important political issue, debated openly in the media. In the general election of 1964, some politicians concentrated on race and immigration as central issues in their campaigns, notably in Smethwick where the Conservative candidate used the slogan, "If you want a nigger neighbour, vote Labour" (Foot, 1965). Labour won the general election, but did not change the immigration policies, and merely shifted its attention to a concern with numbers, advocating integration within immigration controls. They introduced the 1965 Race Relations Act which reduced the number of work vouchers to 8,500 (1,000 of these were for Malta), and established the Race Relations Board which was to begin to look at and act against overt racial discrimination (Hiro, 1973).

The race issue did not come to the fore again until events in East Africa meant that Asians expelled from Kenya could enter Britain under a loophole in the 1962 Act. Enoch Powell declared that, "Hundreds of thousands of people in Kenya, who never dreamt they belonged to this country, started to belong to it like you and me." There was some popular and media support for Powell's fears about the arrival of just over 20,000 people between 1965 and 1967 (Hiro, 1973). The government's reaction was to rush a second Commonwealth Immigrants Act through Parliament in a week in 1968. This Act introduced the distinction between patrials, (those whose parents or grandparents had been born in the UK), who had right of entry and abode, and non-patrials who were no longer allowed in. As a consequence, many white British passport holders living in East Africa could move and settle in the UK, but many Asians could not. There were objections to the Act because of its discriminatory nature, but the Home Secretary, James Callaghan, defended it by declaring that the distinctions were "geographical and not racial."

Also in 1968, the government introduced a second Race Relations Bill. This Bill aimed to extend the powers of the Race Relations Board to challenge overt discrimination in employment, housing, education, entertainment and travel, and to prevent the use of advertisments such as "No coloureds". Opposition to the Bill was substantial, from individuals who would rather go to prison than take down discriminatory notices, from the unions who were against supportive legislation for black workers, from politicians such as Enoch Powell who made his infamous "Rivers of Blood" speech, and from large gatherings of the public in support of Powell's views. The Act was passed, however, and the Community Relations Commission was established. This was followed early in 1969 by the ban on entry of male fiances (Rex and Tomlinson, 1979).

Race and immigration were issues in the 1970 general election. The Tories won, but Edward Heath refused to introduce assistance for repatriation as demanded by Powell. He did, however, introduce an Immigration Bill which was to replace the earlier Aliens Restrictions Acts and Commonwealth Immigrants Acts. When passed, this Immigration Act virtually ended black immigration by restricting the right of residence in the UK to those either born here or whose parents were born here. Again this meant that there was almost free access to immigrants from the Old Commonwealth. Any blacks who did not fit the "patrial" status were allowed in only if they could obtain work permits, which were usually limited to one year and which specified particular jobs (Rees, 1982). These permits were chiefly available for professional occupations, or for jobs which were very poorly paid for long hours, such as NHS ancillary work, or hotel catering and cleaning. The Act also gave greater powers of arrest and deportation of illegal or overstaying immigrants; and made more strict the procedures for the entry of dependants. Women and children could thus be X-rayed on entry to check their ages, some fiancees were subjected to internal examinations to prove their virginity, and intimate and intensive questioning of dependants became routine.

In 1972, immigration became the focus for media attention when Idi Amin threatened to expel several thousand Asians from Uganda. Some 27,000 of these held British passports and so were obliged to come to the UK, rather than to India or Pakistan. Special camps were established for them as they arrived without possessions, and they were urged to settle away from other "Asian" areas to promote integration (Rex and Tomlinson, 1979).

The governments of the 1960s and early 1970s emphasised many times that they were not racist, but that they were concerned for racial integration, assimilation and "good race relations". The Immigration Act sought to limit black immigration, but it did so not by mentioning colour but by emphasising numbers. By 1971, there were 1,151,040 people of New Commonwealth and Pakistan birth in Britain, representing 2.4 per cent of the population. They were largely concentrated in the inner areas of the largest cities, the areas of job opportunity in the 1950s and 1960s.

In the mid 1970s, the government examined the successes and failures of the Race Relations Acts. In 1974, for example, it was found that the Race Relations Board investigated 1,050 cases of claimed racial discrimination. Of these, discrimination was found to be proved in only 224 cases, and of these, 183 were disposed of by conciliation. Eight cases were dropped altogether, and 30 were proceeded with, of which 22 took more than a year to come to court (Jones, 1977). The principal difficulty in all cases was that the discrimination had to be proved conclusively, an almost impossible task unless there were witnesses. The government considered that it should do more, and so in 1976 it introduced a new Race Relations Act with extra powers against people who were "inciting to cause racial hatred". It also established the Commission for Racial Equality (CRE) to replace the Community Relations Commission, and made money available for some black self-help groups. It did not, however, make the passage of complaints any easier. The CRE has been criticised, however, because its upper ranks tend to be dominated by white liberals, and some black groups, such as Race Today, complain that it fails to oppose government policies consistently.

Race emerged again as an issue in the run up to the 1979 general election when the Daily Mail reported a speech of Margaret Thatcher's in which she said: "If we went on as we are now, then by the end of the century there would be four million people of the New Commonwealth and Pakistan here. Now that is an awful lot and I think it means that people are really rather afraid that this country might be swamped by people with a different culture" (cited in Barker, 1981). In 1981, the estimate of people doing the "swamping" was 2,783,000 - 5.2 per cent of the population (OPCS, 1982).

The full relevance of Thatcher's speech is discussed below (Chapter two) but it brought back into consideration what should be done about immigration and the question of repatriation. The 1971 Act had largely ended primary immigration, so the Tories turned their attention to the entry of dependants. The Nationality Act of 1981 was the result. This Act took away the automatic right of citizenship for every person born on British soil - the "ius soli" (Rushdie, 1982). Citizenship was divided into three categories. Full British Citizenship is conferred only on people born in Britain to British citizens, or on people whose parents were born in Britain. British Dependent Territories Citizenship is given to people whose parents are citizens of the Dependent Territories, and they are not allowed free access to the UK. There is also a residual category of British Overseas Citizenship which is conferred on former British passport holders resident in the ex-colonies who did not acquire local citizenship after Independence. Only full British Citizenship confers any rights of entry and abode in the UK, and all other categories must obtain work permits. The holders of British Territories and Overseas Citizenships have very few rights, and the majority of them are black. Consequently, the Act has been termed racist (Ben-Tovim et al, 1982).

The effects of the Nationality Act were quickly felt by black people resident in Britain. Later in 1981, the government introduced a system of charging all people "not normally resident in the UK" for medical treatment. NHS personnel were expected to challenge "likely" non-residents and question them about their place of residence, and amount of time in Britain. Many black people were challenged under this system, the vast majority of whom were legally settled or born in Britain, and after much protest, the system was dropped. Similarly, black Britons have been turned away from French ports when they have tried to enter on one-day passes rather that passports, because customs officials claim that they cannot be sure that blacks are "bona-fide" British citizens. It is against this background that the lives of black people in Britain are set.

THE HISTORY OF RACE RELATIONS/ETHNIC MINORITY STUDIES

Race relations and ethnic minority studies have changed alongside government policy and popular or media-expressed opinion. On the whole, the work has been done by whites, looking at black immigration, cultures, family patterns, employment, housing, education, health and the use of social services. Some of the work has been sponsored by the state; some has been undertaken by state-established concerns such as the CRE; and other work has largely depended upon the dominant ideology or the thinking of contemporary academics or politicians. At first, anthropologists and sociologists studied members of "exotic" cultures as they were discovered by colonialists. As soon as black people arrived in or were brought to Britain and North America, however, they too were studied (Shyllon, 1977). Studies were undertaken to discover how the immigrants lived, how they adapted to life, and what customs they retained (Bourne and Sivanandan, 1980). Mostly, studies have been carried out by white researchers concentrating on the "exotic" and unusual, with very few considering the needs of black people or the effects of personal and institutional racism.

Immigration Studies

Immigration studies have generally taken two forms: they have been concerned either with numbers of immigrants and their locations in Britain, or with the political, economic and social causes and consequences of immigration. The "numbers" studies are generated by the information collected by government agencies such as the Office of

Population and Census Surveys, which publishes and analyses census returns, birth registers, death registers, the International Passenger Survey, and since the late 1970s, the National Dwelling and Housing Survey and the Labour Force Survey (OPCS, 1982a). The numbers of immigrants have been made available by the OPCS itself, the Runnymede Trust, the early work of the Institute of Race Relations, and the CRE.

Individual researchers have used the numbers provided by these organisations as the basis of their work. Peach (1968), for example, discovered that the majority of migrants from the West Indies came to Britain not because they were "pushed" out by population pressure, as earlier studies had suggested, but because they were "pulled" by the perceived job opportunities here. Others have tried to discover the individuals' reasons for migrating by interviewing people in their countries of origin as well as once they have arrived in the UK. Foner (1979) interviewed people in Jamaica and London to uncover their reasons for migrating and their experiences of discrimination in Britain.

Some authors have concentrated on particular immigrant groups or sub-groups in their work: Foner (ibid) on Jamaicans, Philpott (1973) on Montserratians, Anwar (1979) on Pakistanis in Rochdale, and Khan on Asian families (1977) and women (1982). Culture has formed another focus of research on immigrant groups (see Watson, 1977 and Pryce 1979). Much of the research concerning "immigrants" has emphasised their outsider status and looked at the ways in which they have not fitted in to British society and adopted white middle-class norms. Very few studies have been undertaken from the point of view of the people involved, and although racism is acknowledged to be important by Foner (1979) and Khan (in her later work, 1982), it has received scant and insufficient attention.

Employment Studies

The primary reason for the majority of immigrants coming to Britain in the early 1950s and 1960s was to find work (Smith, 1977; Peach, 1968) in response to the needs of British industries after World War II. Some West Indians were recruited directly by organisations such as London Transport and British Rail, and others came to find jobs on the recommendation of friends and relatives. The work that black immigrants obtained was largely confined to the un- or semi-skilled sectors of industries with low rates of pay and poor working conditions. They often took jobs that had been rejected by white workers (Rose, 1969; Brown 1984). In the 1950s, '60s and early '70s, very high proportions of blacks were in employment compared with the whole population, with, for example, 74% of West Indian women working in 1971 compared with 43% of all women (Smith, 1977). Their average earnings, however, tended to be markedly lower than those of whites, and they were under-represented at supervisory levels (Runnymede Trust, 1980).

Black workers tend to be concentrated in the lowest paid industries, the worst conditions and with the least job security (Castles and Kosack, 1973). In 1971, some 47 per cent of black workers were found to be in manufacturing industries compared with only 33 per cent of whites. Black workers also tend to be under-represented in the professional, technical and clerical sectors, even if they have appropriate qualifications - 76 per cent of white men with degrees, for example, are in professional and managerial jobs, compared with only 31 per cent of Asians and Afro-Caribbeans (Smith, 1977). In 1982, 83 per cent of West Indian men and 73 per cent of Asian men, compared with 58 per cent of white men were in manual work (Brown, 1984). Black workers tend also to be concentrated in particular industries such as food, drink and tobacco, metal manufacturing and goods, engineering, vehicles, leather, clothes and footwear, bricks, pottery and cement, and transport (Runnymede Trust, 1980). In London, there are very large numbers of men of Afro-Caribbean descent in transport and labouring jobs; women of Afro-Caribbean descent in the NHS; and people of Asian descent in the service and clothing trades.

Black workers are also over-represented in industries operating shift systems, with 33 per cent of West Indians, 38 per cent of Pakistanis and Bangladeshis working shifts compared with only 14 per cent of whites; and 19 per cent of West Indians and 18 per cent of Pakistanis and Bangladeshis were found to be working permanent night shifts, compared with only nine per cent of whites (Smith, 1977). By 1982, the position was similar, with one third of black men working shifts regularly, compared with one fifth of white men (Brown, 1984). More black women than white also work shifts: 18 per cent of West Indians, 14 per cent of Asians and 11 per cent of whites (Brown, ibid). Despite their long hours and shift work, black workers, particularly men, receive lower wages on average than whites,

The recession of the 1970s and '80s has affected large numbers of workers, particularly those in the manufacturing sector and at the lowest levels of skill. Unemployment doubled in the whole population between 1973 and 1980, but unemployment is much higher among blacks than whites (Runnymede Trust, 1980). The third PSI (Policy Studies Institute) survey found that unemployment was about twice as high among West Indian men and one-and-a-half times as high among Asian men compared with white men (Brown, 1984). For women, unemployment was twice as high for Asians than whites, and one-and-a-half times as high for West Indians than whites. Among black youths, unemployment is particularly severe - perhaps four times as high as among white youths (Hall et al, 1978).

The position of black workers in the most vulnerable industries and at the lowest levels cannot have happened by chance. Racism and other structural factors have combined to produce and reproduce black workers in these positions (Hall et al, 1978). In the PEP (Political and Economic Planning, later re-named Policy Studies Institute) report on racial disadvantage in Britain, Smith (1977) used actors of different ethnic origins to test the existence of deliberate and blatant discrimination. Black and white testers with similar qualifications were sent to apply for jobs, and the white tester was chosen for jobs ten times more often than a black tester, even though the black tester was usually sent out first. Even in letters, it was found that West Indians and Asians faced discrimination in 30% of cases, especially when they applied for junior clerical, accountancy or managerial trainee jobs (Smith, ibid).

The NHS relies heavily on black and immigrant workers brought over on work permits. Black workers comprise one third of hospital medical staff, one fifth of student nurses and midwives, and a very large proportion of ancillary staff. Again, black staff are clearly discriminated against, with large numbers of nurses in the SEN grade rather than the more prestigious SRN grade which allows greater promotion prospects (Doyal, 1980); and overseas doctors being particularly concentrated in junior jobs in the unpopular specialities such as geriatrics, orthopaedics and anaesthetics, with only 12% of them holding the post of consultant compared with 45% of white doctors (Smith, 1980).

Housing Studies

The spatial distribution of black people is closely related to the areas first settled by immigrants in search of job opportunities and relatively cheap accommodation. Areas such as Brick Lane in the east of London have housed generations of immigrants: French Huguenots, East European Jews, and now Bangladeshis. Since the major reason for immigration was to gain employment, the majority have settled and raised their families in metropolitan areas. Estimates from the 1981 census show that 40 per cent of the population of New Commonwealth and Pakistan origin still lives in the Greater London area. Within this area, the black population is concentrated in a few boroughs, especially Hackney, Brent, Newham, Ealing and Lambeth (OPCS, 1982a). In Hackney, for example, 16 per cent of the population is of Afro-Caribbean descent; and in Newham, eight per cent is of Afro-Caribbean and 10 per cent of Asian descent (GLC, 1980).

Housing has been termed the "single most effective cause of racial segregation" (Cottle, 1978). The reasons for the apparent concentration of black people in certain areas are several. Initially, immigrants have tended to take the cheapest and most easily available housing near their jobs and near to people they knew in their countries of origin. Patronage and migration chains have been shown to be of particular importance among Asian settlers (Dahya, 1974; Anwar, 1979). Groups of people of similar ethnic origin may also prefer to come together for cohesion and to enable them to retain important cultural and religious practices (Lee, 1977). There is evidence to suggest, however, that racial discrimination is also an important factor.

According to Rose (1969), Smith (1977), the Runnymede Trust (1980) and Brown (1984), black people fare worse than whites in almost all types of housing. Although large numbers of people of Asian origin own their own homes, they tend to have much lower quality properties than whites: only 16 per cent of black people own detached houses compared with 57 per cent of whites; 66 per cent of blacks compared with 30 per cent of whites own terraced houses; and twice the number of blacks as whites own pre-1914 properties (Smith, 1977). This may be the result of choice, socio-economic status, or a reflection of the properties available in the inner city areas settled by black people, but it seems likely that racial discrimination is also involved.

Table 1(i): Housing Tenure According to Race of Head of Household

	Owner Occupied	Rented from Local Authority	Private rented unfurnished	Private rented furnished
West Indian	35%	52%	6%	7%
Asian	62%	16%	8%	13%
White	45%	34%	15%	6%

(National Dwelling and Household Survey, 1977-8)

The private housing market offers many opportunities for racial discrimination, and before the 1968 Race Relations Act, it was not uncommon to see signs such as "No Coloureds" outside homes for sale or rent. Asians have been most successful in buying their own homes, sometimes obtaining mortgages, other times buying them outright as family groups. It would seem from evidence in Handsworth that they have had mainly to rely on bank loans and council mortgages to buy property (Rex and Tomlinson, 1979), perhaps because the houses have been in poor condition or in unpopular, inner city areas, some of which may have been due for demolition. West Indians have tended not to buy their own homes in such large numbers (see Table 1(i)), and they, like whites, seem to have relied upon building societies and councils for their mortgages (Rex and Tomlinson, ibid). Building societies and estate agents have some power over housing allocation, and some degree of racial segregation in the private market may be due to agents who show black customers only those houses in areas thought to be "suitable" - the inner cities rather than suburbia (Lee, 1977). Or it may be that members of ethnic groups prefer the inner cities (Dahya, 1974) - the assumption that suburban semis are best may be a white, middle-class conception.

In local authority housing, black people fare very badly. Newly arrived immigrants do not fit the three to five year "resident in the borough" qualification often necessary to go onto the housing waiting list, and consequently, they get allocated emergency housing, usually in very poor condition or on the least popular estates. In the late 1970s, the GLC admitted that the residential qualifications discriminate against immigrants, but blame this on the operation of procedures rather than on active discrimination (Smith, 1977). It is not only immigrants who suffer. Another study of GLC housing allocations showed that black people were under-represented in council accommodation, and that they were much more likely to be in pre-1914 flats in central London than whites (Runnymede Trust, 1980). The third PSI survey also showed that the council properties occupied by black people are, overall, markedly inferior to those occupied by whites: blacks live in smaller, more crowded properties; are more likely to be in flats than houses and on higher floors; and they rarely have access to gardens (Brown, 1984). It was also found that one quarter of black tenants had applied for a transfer to another property, compared with less than one eighth of white tenants (Brown, ibid).

The GLC has over the last few years, handed over the organisation of its housing to the boroughs, and several of these are investigating their allocation procedures with a view to altering their policies to prevent discrimination against black tenants. A recent report from Hackney, for example, showed that although one half of the people on the council lists are black, only 21 per cent of blacks were offered houses compared with 79 per cent of whites; only 12 per cent of blacks were offered new property compared with 88 per cent of whites; 75 per cent of blacks got pre-war property compared with 25 per cent of whites; and on the housing estate considered by local residents to be the "worst" in terms of amenities, safety and environmental quality, one half of the tenants were black, although they make up only 24 per cent of the tenants of Hackney (CRE, 1984). The report concluded that its new policies to ignore residential qualifications and to help black tenants were being thwarted by active racial discrimination by staff in the housing department.

In the private renting market, all tenants are at potential risk from unscrupulous land and property owners. Higher rents for black tenants in multi-occupied, old houses rarely maintained or repaired have been found (Smith, 1977; Lee, 1977). According to Rose (1969), some 70 per cent of all households with a New Commonwealth or Pakistani head in London were sharing accommodation, and in 1982, it was found that 17 per cent of West Indian households, 44 per cent of Asian households compared with 1 per cent of white households had housing densities of more than one person per room (Brown, 1984). Unlike the study in the late 1960s, however, the most recent PSI survey found that levels of amenities were not affected by race so much as by tenure and area of residence. The lack of amenities in more black households than white was more a function of the greater number of blacks in poor quality rented accommodation in inner city areas than in owner-occupied suburbia (Brown, 1984). Moving away from the deprived and increasingly derelict inner cities may be one way for black people to improve their housing, but while building societies, estate agents and local authorities may discriminate against them, such "dispersal" even if it is desired, is likely to be only minimal.

Dispersal of black tenants has been tried in Wolverhampton, where the local authority operated a policy of housing "coloured" families at least five doors away from their nearest "coloured" neighbour, or ensuring that there was only one "coloured" family per two floors of any block of flats (Deakin, 1970). Problems arose as to who was "coloured", and the policy became unworkable. Whether or not dispersal is a good policy is open to argument, especially, as Lee (1977) points out, it cannot be assumed that spatial dispersal will result in social integration (the policy aim), because the two things are not necessarily related.

Education

The education system reflects the dominant sub-culture of society - white, Anglo-Saxon and Protestant - and it is imbued with middle-class values, assumptions and expectations (Khan, 1982). The number of black teachers is minimal, being less than 5% of all teachers, and there is evidence to suggest that these are restricted to certain areas and low pay scales (Runnymede Trust, 1980). The numbers of black children, however, are substantial, although estimated to be only 3.3% of all school children in 1971. The black population is young in comparison to the white majority: some 30 per cent of West Indians and 40 per cent of Asians are aged between 0 and 16 years, compared with 22 per cent of the whole population in 1981. In some areas, black pupils make up very high proportions of the school population - up to 80 or 90 per cent in some schools in Spitalfields, London.

The response of schools to black children has typically involved the labelling of children as "problems" (Carby, 1982a). Early policy was to assimilate the children into the system, to absorb them, hoping that the children would change. When this failed, the "problems" were shifted away from the children and onto black culture or family patterns (Carby, ibid). Educational testing, for example, "proved" the lower IQs of black children, although ignoring the ethnocentricity of the tests. The key was seen to be learning standard English, and so all other language speakers were given extra tuition in English as a second language. This was not so for the West Indian children, whose language was thought to be an "immature" or "deviant" form of English, rather than a completely separate dialect with different syntax and word constructions (Lawrence, 1982b).

Another focus of concern for the educational system was the "culture" of black children which was thought to hamper their progress. Writers such as Pryce (1979), suggest that West Indian children are "severely handicapped" because of their mutilating colonial heritage. Not everyone now agrees with him (see CCCS, 1982). Dispersal of black children was suggested in 1963, with black children being bussed to outlying schools to prevent the numbers of black children rising too high in some schools. This policy was not officially ended until 1978, and again it emphasised the location of the "problems" within the black community. Meanwhile, Coard (1971) discovered that although West Indian children were only 1.1 per cent of all children, they were 5 per cent of the children in schools for the educationally sub-normal. Other writers began to look at the content of school books, and discovered that racism was an important force acting against black children in schools.

Journals such as the New Statesman and Contemporary Issues in Geography and Education have monitored and exposed racist or ethnocentric books. Textbooks such as Young and Lowry's Regions of the World, reprinted many times, and Davies', Problems Around Us, have been labelled as racist and their use discouraged (Hicks, 1982; Wright, 1983). Teachers' attitudes to pupils are also of importance in influencing children's performances (Rose, 1969), and there have been many reports of teachers who espouse racist views, who cannot look black children in the eye or who refuse physical contact with them in PE (Cottle, 1978; Gill, 1983).

The latest policy initiative of the DES is multi-cultural education. This requires teachers to inform pupils about cultures other than their own, and aims to treat all cultures equally. It tends, therefore, to ignore the power relations in society. Children may now have lessons in Asian cookery and learn some black dub poetry, but the training of teachers has been very patchy, and the policy's implementation has been largely restricted to the more progressive, inner city schools (Carby, 1982a). Some black people see multi-culturalism as yet another decoy from racism (Sivanandan, 1983; Carby, 1982a), and advocate a policy of more thorough anti-racist teaching in all schools, not just those with large numbers of black pupils. As it stands, the education system, even with its multi-cultural teaching, serves to preserve and re-inforce the dominant ideology and discriminatory nature of British society.

Women and the Family

The "family", has provided a particular focus for "ethnic" research, and vast generalisations and assumptions abound in this work about the (stereo-)typical black family (Lawrence, 1982b). Afro-Caribbean families are seen to be matriarchal in structure, often having only one parent, with mothers who work, and a general lack of discipline because of the assumed absence of a strong male presence (Lawrence, ibid; Parmar, 1982). The evidence for much of this work has come from the Moynihan Report (see Rainwater and Yancy, 1967), which was the result of studies of black families in the USA, and which propounded the theory of the "tangle of pathology" within black American families. Asian families, on the other hand, are seen to be patriarchal in structure, with a dominating male presence, a submissive mother, usually living in overcrowded housing and with inter-generational conflicts (Allen, 1982; Parmar, 1982; Carby, 1982). Such assumptions are imbued with the conception of the "ideal" family type of two (married) adults and one or two children, and there is a marked tendency to see other family patterns as deviant, even pathological, without considering the reasons for the patterns or the possibility that they too may have advantages.

It is a short step from seeing black families in these "deviant" terms to blaming them for what are considered to be the "problems" of the black community. Hence the Centre for Contemporary Cultural Studies (1982) cites research which blames the myth of violent and criminal black youth, high rates of child accidents, and low levels of educational achievement on the make-up of Afro-Caribbean families. This has been particularly true in the case of black youth, where the assumed lack of family discipline and absence of a male presence, is seen to be the reason for young black men turning to crime and young women turning to promiscuity and inevitable pregnancy (Hall et al, 1978; Gilroy, 1982). Writers such as Pryce (1979), Driver (1982) and Evans (1971) have been accused of perpetuating these views by presenting these stereotypes in their work.

For Asian families, the reaction has been somewhat different. There have been assumptions that overcrowding may be a consequence of the extended family; and in particular that there are conflicts between parents and their children over the subject of arranged marriages (Lawrence, 1982a; Parmar, 1982). Writers such as Khan, in her early work (1977), and Ballard (1982) have been accused of helping to perpetuate the stereotypes of the rigid rules in Asian families and the supposed submissiveness of Asian women (Parmar, 1982; Allen, 1982).

There have also been many assumptions about the status of black women in race relations research. White feminists have attacked the unequal power held by men in society, but they have assumed that all women's experience of patriarchy is the same. Slavery and imperialism, however, have denied black men the authoritarian positions held by white men, and so black women's experience of patriarchy has been different (Carby, 1982b). Consequently, white women have seen themselves as free and liberated, but have seen Asian women as isolated and enclosed, and Afro-Caribbean women as workers who let their children run wild (Carby, ibid).

During the time of slavery in the US and Britain, Afro-Caribbean women had an ambiguous role. Unlike Afro-Caribbean men, they were seen as docile, and so were allowed to look after white children, but at the same time they were exploited sexually by white men (Lerner, 1972). Lerner (ibid), cites work that shows the rarely-studied examples of black-American women's continual struggles against white society, by shamming illness, resisting orders, and influencing the white children in their care. After slavery, even though their lot was arduous and restricted, the family has been the focus of resistance, with black women playing a crucial role, and it would appear that the fight against racial discrimination has always been seen to be more important than the fight against sexism (Lerner, ibid).

Asian women have been even less visible in race relations studies. As indicated above, they tend to be seen as submissive, passive and silent, and very few studies have considered their experiences of migration and/or working in Britain. Asian women often have to work very long hours in the Third World, where among kinship groups purdah may not inhibit their working outside, but in Britain, they are considered to be non-workers (Parmar, 1982). Asian women, when they do work here, tend to be confined to very low paid jobs such as home machining, laundry, electronics assembly, cleaning and canteen work - all jobs for which they are, no doubt, considered "suitable" according to the conception employers have of them. Similarly, it has been shown that Asian girls may not be given adequate advice for careers in further education because careers are deemed to be "inappropriate" (Lawrence, 1982a). These ideas of Asian women's passivity and submissiveness seem to persist despite their publicised struggles at Grunwick in 1977, and in the East End of London under the title of the Sari Squad in 1983-4. These publicised struggles hide a plethora of others.

<u>Health and the Social Services</u>

Accusations have often been levelled at newly arrived immigrants that they are less healthy and hygienic than the population as a whole

(Jones, 1977). Consequently, information about, and figures of, the utilization of the health and welfare services by immigrants and their descendants have been, and still are, political issues. Fears that immigrants will bring in, or cause the spread of conditions such as tuberculosis, VD, leprosy and so on have been raised by the public and researchers (see Donovan, 1984), and they have emerged periodically during general elections (Foot, 1965). These ideas neglect the fact that the majority of immigrants work hard, and that they pay taxes and National Insurance, thus fully entitling them to social and health services.

In the USA, the experience of health is clearly divided along racial lines. Minorities in the US are three times as likely as whites to die of hypertension, four times as likely to die of kidney problems, twice as likely to die of diabetes, and five times as likely to die of TB (from the Civil Rights Digest, 1977, cited by eds. Contemp. Issues in Geog. and Education, 1984). In 1977, there were 80,000 more black deaths than expected compared with white deaths, and a 90% excess of infant deaths among blacks compared with whites (Cooper, 1983). As Cooper says, "Race is a powerful determinant of health" (ibid, 5), but not because of any genetic or biological factors. It is the effects of racism and the workings of capitalism that are to be blamed (Cooper, ibid).

In Britain, figures for the health status and use of health services by minority groups have not been kept so thoroughly as in the US, and so much of the "evidence" about black people's health is patchy and inconclusive. The Black Report (DHSS, 1980a), although the most detailed analysis of health in Britain to date, virtually ignored black people, claiming that there was too little adequate information. What research has been done has focused on the "exotic" diseases such as cholera, TB, yaws and so on which are thought to have been brought in by immigrants; or on conditions that are thought to affect particular groups such as thalassaemia. These are all considered in more detail in chapter three.

Conclusion

The history of British imperialism and immigration impinges upon the lives of black people today. On an international scale, neo-colonialism contrives to dominate trading between the developed and under-developed worlds and to perpetuate the unequal relationships between rich and poor countries (see Rodney, 1972). In Britain, images of the imperialist past and the unequal present remain. Legislation has virtually put a stop to immigration, but it has not yet started to tackle the racial discrimination that pervades all aspects of the state and influences individuals.

The workings of the economic and urban systems have tended to confine black people to the worst paid, dirtiest and most dangerous jobs, and restricted them to the worst housing and environmental conditions. Racial discrimination has played a crucial role in the economic and political position of black workers, because it creates stereotypes which inform employers, estate agents and so on about what jobs and houses are "suitable" for black people. The report on the health of the nation, although largely ignoring black people, documented clearly the links between class and health (DHSS, 1980a; Townsend and Davidson, 1982). It showed, for example, that Classes IV and V (the manual workers, skilled and unskilled), fare worse on almost all indices of health and illness than those in Classes I and II (the professional and managerial workers) (DHSS, ibid). Since it has been shown that a large proportion of the black community has been confined to Classes IV and V, (see Allen and Smith, 1974; Phizacklea and Miles, 1980) it may be assumed that their health is likely to be as poor as the whites in these same classes.

At different times, different "solutions" have been proposed to black "problems", but rarely have black people been consulted. Policies have changed superficially from a concern that black people should be assimilated into the majority white society, to multiculturalism, which propounds the view that all cultures should be retained on an equal basis. Below the surface, however, the policies have changed very little, and racism has escaped and is still escaping largely unchallenged. The typical tendency for researchers has been to "blame the victim", and to see black people as "the problem", or at least having lots of "problems." Racism, and its effects have either been measured but then ignored by successive governments (see Smith, 1977); or buried within the "more powerful" class relations (see Phizacklea and Miles, 1980). Sometimes they have been ignored altogether. Too often immigration, ethnic minority and multi-cultural studies have ignored the real root of the issue, racism, and become caught up in the debate about the primacy of race or culture.

2 Race or culture: the debate

Studies of ethnic groups and race relations in Britain have tended to polarise into two schools; one has concentrated on "culture" and its effects; and the other has focused on minority status and the importance of racism. The former school draws particularly upon anthropological and sociological work; the latter more on politics and economics. Both schools experience difficulties in definition: the cultural school over what "culture" consists of, particularly how it differs from "society", and how it affects behaviour; the race school over the concept of "race", and an adequate definition of racism. In the area of health studies, the polarisation of the two schools has tended to lead to the neglect of important overlaps and similarities. It is the purpose of this chapter to describe the cultural view in detail, to consider the importance of the race view as outlined in chapter one, and to assess the relevance of the two views in a study of black people's health.

"CULTURE"

Culture, according to the Oxford English Dictionary (1964), is merely, "intellectual development". In the Penguin English Dictionary (1965), it is the, "state of intellectual, artistic and social development of a group ... [the] type and degree of civilization." Kroeber and Kluckholm (in the International Encyclopaedia of the Social Sciences, 1968, 528) give a much wider definition: culture, they maintain, includes:

> "Patterns, explicit and implicit, of and for behaviour acquired and transmitted by symbols, constituting the distinctive achievement of human groups, including their embodiment in artefacts; the essential core of culture consists of tradition (ie historically derived and selected) ideas and especially their attached values; culture systems may, on the one hand, be considered as a product of action, on the other as conditioning elements of further action."

The sociological definition of culture in the Fontana Dictionary of Modern Thought (1977, 150) is even wider and all-encompassing: culture is:

> "The 'social heritage' of a community: the total body of material artefacts (tools, weapons, houses; places of work, worship, government, recreation; works of art etc), of collective mental and spiritual 'artefacts' (systems of symbols, ideas, beliefs, aesthetic perceptions, values etc), and of distinctive forms of behaviour (institutions, groupings, rituals, modes of organisation etc) created by a people (sometimes deliberately, sometimes through unforseen interconnections and consequences) in their on-going activities within their particular life-conditions, and (though undergoing kinds and degrees of change) transmitted from generation to generation."

Individual writers define culture in many different ways, and there apppears to be considerable confusion over what is "cultural" and what is "social", as well as whether or not there is any differentiation between the two.

A medical sociologist, Mechanic, sees culture as designating "a totality of inter-related but often disjointed and contradictory ideas and activities that characterise the way of life of a particular social group" (1978, 35). Saunders, however, feels that culture consists of a "vast complex of knowledge, beliefs, techniques, roles, norms, values, ideologies, attitudes, customs, rituals and symbols that interlock to form a mutually re-inforcing and supporting system" (1954, 7). On the whole, more medical sociologists would seem to agree with Saunders that culture is a complex system, even a "whole way of life" (Susser and Watson, 1971, 42). The idea of culture being a "system", however, may have emerged in part because of the ideas of a powerful school of sociology, the structural-functionalists, who tend to see society and its constituent parts in terms of systems or subsystems (see, for example, Parsons, 1951).

Although they disagree over a precise definition of the concept of culture, medical sociologists are in agreement over the important effects it has upon perceptions and behaviour. "Culture" involves the beliefs and customs a society develops in attempting to manage its shared problems (Enos and Sultan, 1977), and orders "proper" behaviour, priorities, social norms and values (Twaddle and Hessler, 1977). It is embodied in language, the primary form of communication (Fabrega and Tyma, 1976), subtly and systematically affects perception (Paul, 1955), and invests it with emotional significance (Hsu, 1955). Culture is not always explicit, and may not necessarily be recognised by individuals (Paul, 1955), but it is of particular importance because it can be transmitted through generations (Mechanic, 1978), and thus cause the persistance of certain behaviours that may appear to be anachronistic.

In general terms, then, culture refers to the historical development of a group of people, and consists of their "recipes" for living in the world. These "recipes" are explored further in chapter four (see also Schutz, 1972). Parts of culture, such as patterns of diet and clothing, may be tenaciously held by some people at some times, but they may also be changed by new information or in response to perceived threats or desires. Culture is, therefore, a mixture of the static and variable, depending on external and internal pressures for stability and change. Some members of minority groups such as Sikhs in Britain, for example, may retain practices seen to be pivotal to their cultures such as the reluctance to cut hair, but may feel able to drop other habits which may not fit in with the majority society, such as the carrying of daggers. Some Sikhs in Britain have found it necessary to stop wearing turbans in order to further their careers. Hostility from the majority society may result in the resurrection of cultural practices or the growth of new beliefs from old ideas, such as the development of Hasidism among Jews and Rastafarianism among Afro-Caribbean youths. Culture is, therefore, an important, but very complex factor in people's lives.

CULTURE AND HEALTH

According to anthropological and sociological literature, culture affects the perceptions of health and illness, and the responses to episodes of ill-health. Culture is assumed to mediate between the individual and the environment (Paul, 1955), and to establish rules and norms governing what an illness is and the appropriate responses to different episodes (Lewis, 1981). Culture may affect the ways in which biological changes in the body will be perceived and acted upon (or not), depending upon expectations, taboos and current levels of knowledge about causes and effects (Pfifferling, 1981). The experience and expression of symptoms may also be influenced by culture (Good and Good, 1981), as may be the amount of information a patient elects to give to a medical practitioner (Enos and Sultan, 1977). Similarly, the duration of a condition will be delimited by expectations and cultural knowledge (Susser and Watson, 1971). Thus it is claimed that culture establishes guides for individuals which enable them to know when they or others may be regarded as ill; it discloses something about the causes and nature of particular episodes of ill-health and what should be done about them; and it delimits the behaviour expected of individuals who are given the label "ill" or "sick" (Saunders, 1954).

Some studies have been undertaken to look at the effects of culture on health. Some writers have focused on health and illness among "primitive" groups such as the inhabitants of Yap, a Pacific island (Schneider, 1955). Others have studied people with "exotic" cultures, such as the Taiwanese (Kleinman, Eisenberg and Good, 1978), and the inhabitants of Trinidad and Tobago (Aho and Minott, 1977). Similarly, there are studies of health and illness among distinctive ethnic groups within "developed" societies: blacks, Mexican Americans and American Indians (Enos and Sultan, 1977); Spanish Americans (Saunders, 1954); and West Indians in Britain (Patterson, 1963; Kiev, 1963). These studies all tend to emphasise the exotic and unusual elements of the individuals' cultures, and focus on the negative effects (as they are seen by western eyes) that their cultural practices may have on their health. This "bias" in ethnicity and health literature is explored further in chapter three.

Culture, Health and Illness

The concept of "health" is wide-ranging. According to the WHO, it is, "a state of complete physical, mental and social well-being, and not merely the absence of disease and infirmity." This all-embracing statement relies, however, on common sense conceptions of normality and well-being (Dingwall, 1976). Health is sometimes seen as a "norm" or an ideal (Brearley, 1978), but others would suggest that it may be that having some symptoms is the "healthy" norm (Zola, 1975a). Some claim that health is intimately connected with the way people construct social reality (Nader and Maretzki, 1973), and their experiences in everyday life. Hence Robinson, (1971), found that tiredness was accepted as part of life by some of the working class people he studied, whereas it was considered to be indicative of illness among some of the middle-class respondents. The concept of health is intricately tied to an individual's cultural conceptions of normality. Typically, health is seen as a residual category - the absence of illness or infirmity rather than anything specific, and writers go on to consider illness and disease in much greater detail.

Illness tends to be differentiated from disease in medical sociology. Illness is considered to be a perceptual category, whereas disease is a biological malfunction. Illness may be the perception of a condition of impaired well-being (Helman, 1978), or a state of psychic awareness of discomfort (Susser and Watson, 1971), or the subjective and psychological dimension of non-health (Twaddle, 1981). To be more precise, illness is a state created by individuals to give meaning to their experience of symptoms and disease (Locker, 1981) and it is presumed to be a personal category, bounded by cultural and social norms. According to Parsons (1951) illness should be considered to be a state of deviance because it prevents individuals from fulfilling their economic and social obligations.

Disease, however, is not affected by perception: it is, according to Western and scientific medicine, a clinically-defined abnormality in the structure or function of body systems (Eisenberg and Kleinman, 1981). It is thus a state of physical or psychological dysfunction (Susser and Watson, 1971), or the pathological process underlying the clinical syndrome (Mechanic, 1978). As such, it is quite different from the concept of illness. Although diseases are the biological dimension of non-health (Twaddle, 1981), they are positively or negatively viewed according to social and cultural norms (Brody, 1981). In most societies, illness and disease are extremely closely tied. It may be possible, for example, for illness to be perceived where no disease can be discovered, or where symptoms persist after a condition is thought to have been cured; and disease may exist without illness having been perceived, as, for example, in cancer patients who do not feel any different. It has also been suggested that "patients suffer illness; doctors diagnose and treat disease" (Eisenberg, 1977, 9), because of the gulf between lay perceptions and professional judgements (see below).

Sickness is sometimes separately defined as the social dimension of ill-health, or the state in which an individual cannot fulfil her/his social obligations. A classic work in this field is Parsons' conception of the "sick role". According to Parsons, illness should be considered to be a form of deviance because it causes an individual to withdraw from social life (1951). Illness is thus a threat to the established social order, and so some form of social control becomes essential to maintain the steady state of society. Consequently, sick individuals are obliged to take up, temporarily, the "sick role". They are isolated from fellow sufferers and are expected to get well, but they are also exempted from their social duties, are not blamed for their condition, and are obliged to consult a doctor who is assumed by Parsons to be an altruistic and neutral practitioner of the benign medical system (Parsons, 1951).

This interpretation of the response to ill-health has been criticised and exposed for being culturally and historically specific, reflecting as it does the Protestant work ethic and the approach of the structural-functionalist branch of sociological theory (Fabrega, 1977; Ehrenreich, 1978). These authors and others have also criticised Parsonian theory for asserting that medicine is a benign system and its practitioners neutral. Medicine has been seen by others as being dominated by professionalism (Freidson, 1970a, 1973); the cause of more illness than it can cure (Illich, 1976); an instrument of social control (Zola, 1975b; Ehrenreich, 1978); and an instrument of capitalism and the state (Navarro, 1978). (These views are considered in greater depth, below).

Perceptions of Ill-Health

Any change in the body state that is not considered to be "normal" may be perceived as an illness. The identification of a condition depends in the first place upon an individual's conception of normal (Mechanic, 1978). Normality is generally assumed to be defined and delimited by cultural factors, which use past experience and present conditions to assess typical occurrences and to label any deviations "illness". Perception is an intensely personal feeling, in which the world is experienced and given meaning (Lewis, 1981). According to Kohn and White, (1976, 11), perception:

> "Constitutes man's [sic] capacity to receive and communicate information - ie symptoms - from the psychobiological system, to compare it with information from the external social system and with information stored in his [sic] memory, and to detect imbalance."

This imbalance is then assessed to see if it fits the category of illness.

Imbalances and changes in the state of the body are usually perceived initially as symptoms. These are perceived and defined according to culturally accepted limits (Twaddle and Hessler, 1977). As Mechanic says, "Symptoms are differentially perceived, evaluated and acted upon (or not acted upon) by different kinds of people and in different situations" (1978, 249). This may reflect the magnitude, quality, seriousness or severity of the symptoms themselves, or may be due to cultural factors which may consider ubiquitous symptoms to be "normal", or social factors which may consider certain symptoms to be unimportant on some occasions but crucial on others.

Some sufferers may perceive some symptoms or illnesses as a threat, punishment, enemy, relief or strategy (Pfifferling, 1981), depending on the social context (or cultural history). A set of symptoms may be immediately perceived as an illness in some cultures, but ignored as part of life in others - such as the acceptance of blood in urine by people living in areas of endemic schistosomiasis. Fear and anxiety may also affect the perception of symptoms as illness. Fear of cancer, for example, may lead to individuals denying to themselves that they have any symptoms at all. Stress, according to Kleinman (1980), may lead to the somatisation of complaints - the expression of worries and mental tensions as physical conditions. Somatisation may also occur where patients find it difficult to communicate with doctors, when physical symptoms may be much easier to explain.

There have been studies in the US of cultural differences in the perception of pain. Zborowski, for example, (1952 and cited in Cox and Mead, 1975; Stoeckle and Barsky, 1981), studied the reactions of members of the Irish, Italian, Jewish and Old American ethnic groups to pain in hospital. He claimed that Irish respondents concentrated particularly on problems located in the eyes, ears, nose or throat, but avoided complaining specifically of pain; whereas Italians and Jews were supposed to be very expressive about pain, and to complain about pains in various locations. Old Americans were found to be very "stoical". Zborowski also claimed that Italians were concerned particularly with the need for immediate pain relief, whereas Jews were worried about the long term consequences of the pain, and Old Americans and Irish were neutral. In similar sorts of studies, Zola (1975a) and Twaddle and Hessler (1977), supported these findings.

In these studies, the reactions of Old Americans in particular and the Irish are viewed favourably. Their reactions are described as "stoical" and "neutral", and are considered to be normal. The others, however, are seen to be "very expressive", and to complain about pains that may not exist. It may be that the individuals' responses to pain are culturally determined, but there is a bias in the studies that tends to label the behaviour of non-Anglo-Saxons inappropriate. The reactions of medical staff to patients who are members of ethnic groups may also be important (Dingwall, 1976). These issues are further explored in chapter three.

Fig.2(i) Diagrammatic Representation of Pathways to Care

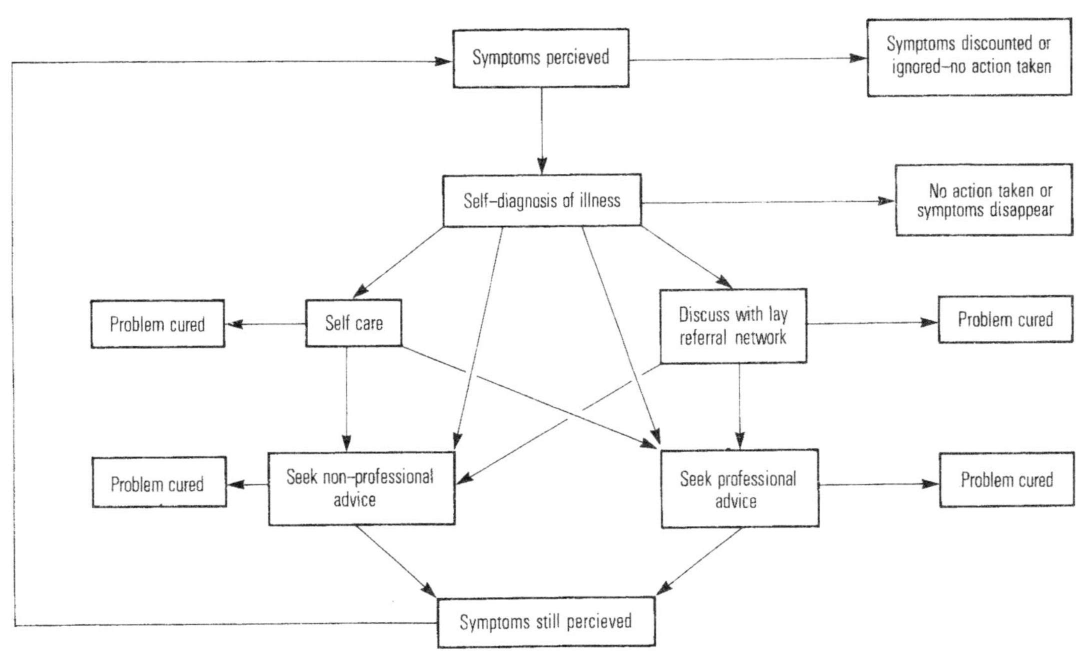

Responses to Ill-Health

Once a set of symptoms has been perceived to be an illness, individuals have to choose between a selection of possible actions (see Figure 2(i)). There is a pathway to care, for example, from the perception of a problem, through the defining of it as such, to attempts to seek care (Rosenstock, 1966). This pathway is not the only response, however. On many occasions, symptoms will be perceived, only to be discounted as normal or ignored, either because they are thought or hoped to be unimportant, or because to admit them and to take further action may interfere with economic and social obligations. There is an initial period, therefore, of self-diagnosis and assessment for symptoms that are not visible to others (Eisenberg, 1980). This period will be the time in which the condition will be compared with previous experience and the expectations arising from these.

The perceived severity of the condition is thought to be of particular importance, as measured by the form, duration and intensity of symptoms and the restrictions these impose on normal activities (Kohn and White, 1976; Enos and Sultan, 1977). It may be that the interference with daily life by a set of symptoms may be the major criterion of ill-health (McKinlay, 1981). The self-diagnosis that ill-health is present does not necessarily lead the sufferer straight to health-care services. In fact, some 75 to 90 per cent of all self-diagnosed illnesses are thought to be dealt with outside the professional sphere (Kleinman, Eisenberg and Good, 1977).

If symptoms are visible to others, or if a person has decided that she/he is suffering from some sort of ill-health, reference will usually be made to other family members to elicit their opinions and advice. Other relatives or friends may also be included in the discussions, and these form the lay referral system (Kohn and White, 1976). This "popular" sector of health care may provide remedies, discount the symptoms as unimportant, pass the person on to another member of the network thought to be better qualified, or advise a consultation with some sort of healing practitioner. If symptoms persist or worsen after self and/or lay treatment or advice, the help of outsiders is likely then to be employed. In many cases, this is very much a last resort (Brearley, 1978).

The existence, extent and competence of lay networks varies by social class, ethnicity and individual factors. It is believed that the middle- and upper-classes, with their longer education, tend to share similar beliefs and values with the medical profession, and so they have little need for a lay network at all (Freidson, 1973; Mechanic, 1978). Where people's values differ from those of the medical profession, lay networks are likely to exist and persist, based usually upon kinship and friendship patterns, or within minority and cultural groups (Mechanic, ibid). In a study of white, working- and middle-class people, Helman (1978), found that the amount of self diagnosis and lay treatment varied according to class and factors such as loneliness, widowhood and stress. People with few friends or relatives nearby, and people who suffer from a lot of stress are supposed to have very limited networks, and to rely heavily on the professional health services (Wadsworth, 1971; Pilisuk and Froland, 1978). It has been suggested that strong networks may lead to individuals suffering fewer illnesses (McKinlay, 1981), although it is not clear which is the cause and which the effect.

Since such a large proportion of ill-health is dealt with outside the professional sector, it would appear that an individual must, in general, perceive a condition to be quite serious before arranging a consultation with a GP. Access may also be of importance, as although in Britain, everybody is supposed to have equal and free access to health-care, physical distance, lack of a 'phone, inability to take time off work, and the demands of child-care may all impede access to physicians. Fear of the result of the consultation may also delay visits. For many reasons, then, GPs see only the "tip of the iceberg" of people's illnesses and diseases (Hannay, 1979).

Lay and Professional Antagonisms

Healers in most cultures are seen to be of high status. This has been particularly so in the case of modern medicine, where members of the hierarchically-arranged medical profession are drawn almost exclusively from the ranks of the upper- and middle-classes. They are also largely white and male, thus forming almost a cultural minority themselves (Pfifferling, 1981). Science is imbued with ideas about neutrality, superiority and rationality, and so the medical profession, with its scientific background, has come to dominate the health-care field and other spheres of life. In this century, medicine has extended its interest into alcoholism, drug-taking and now plays a major role in legal cases where insanity is claimed or suspected. Illich (1976) has termed medicine a radical monopoly, because of its tendency to take over whatever comes within its grasp.

Illich has undertaken a thorough critique of modern scientific medicine (1976). He sees it as an all-embracing system of social control, which unlike practices of healing at other times, is capable of causing actual harm to patients through iatrogenesis. This iatrogenesis takes three forms: clinical, in which harm is done directly in the clinical encounter; social, in which people's lay beliefs are superseded by low levels of tolerance to pain and they become increasingly dependent upon physicians; and cultural, which has destroyed traditional ways of coping with illness and death, forcing people into believing that they need more and more medical care. There are flaws in Illich's analysis. He discounts, for example, the possibility that medicine, through public health, has ever done anything but harm people's health, yet advances in public health and hygiene clearly wiped out many endemic diseases (McKeown, 1976). Illich also harks back to the halcyon days of some imaginary era when everybody took care of their own health - a time that has clearly never been; and he sees people today as being bereft of any ability to look after themselves, and as fearful, acquiescent victims.

The scientific training of doctors, coupled with their elite and privileged status, means that they are somewhat divorced from the majority of people they treat. Their training inculcates the idea that "their" medicine is right, rational and absolute, and that lay beliefs are largely inconsistent, partially clear, irrational and untestable (Dingwall, 1976). Their expectations and values may be different from those of their patients: hence doctors complain of people who fill their surgeries with "trivial" conditions (Wadsworth, 1971); or who arrive too late for anything to be done for them (Paul, 1955). Freidson (1970a, 1970b) argues that the medical profession has obtained exclusive jurisdiction over determining what an illness is and how it should be recognised. He sees "professional dominance" as a major obstacle to good health care, but he also sees the "lower" classes as being ignorant and having out-dated and antiquated ideas.

It is important for doctors to realise that the expressed demand for health-care which they see in their surgeries is only the final outcome of a period of intensive self-diagnosis, lay referral, or consultation with non-registered practitioners such as herbalists, chiropractors and homeopaths. Appearance at a surgery or outpatients department also means that the individual is likely to have balanced the costs (financial and social) of visiting a physician against the expected outcome of the visit (Kohn and White, 1976). Thus the patient may bring to the encounter a vast array of pre-conceived ideas, worries and possible solutions to their health problems, and these views may not necessarily be shifted by what a physician has to say.

These differences between sufferer and carer may well result in the apparent non-compliance of the sufferer, especially if the carer fails to understand the patient's background and anxieties (Zola, 1981). Hence in this study, several women of Asian descent do not take the recommended number of pills prescribed by their doctors because they feel that more than one pill a day will affect the balance of the body, and because more than one pill makes them feel "hot". Instances of non-compliance are likely to be more common where the backgrounds of patients and physicians are most different (Susser and Watson, 1971; Mechanic, 1978; Kleinman, 1980).

Some writers, such as Parsons (1951), assume that the clinical encounter between a physician and a patient is equal. Others claim that the differences in class and status of the two means that in any consultation, the physician will normally hold the power and tend to operate as an instrument of social control (Ehrenreich, 1978; Zola, 1975b), or the servant of the capitalist state (Navarro, 1978). The power of medicine can be seen in the "medicalisation of life" - the way it interferes with and often dominates many spheres of life. Its power tends to reflect and re-inforce the dominant ideology and the status quo, and it has largely excluded women and minority groups. It has similarly excluded and belittled lay views of health and illness.

RACE OR CULTURE : THE DEBATE

Much of the research on health and illness has been concerned with the effects of "culture". Culture has been seen to have an influential effect on perceptions of health and illness, conceptions of normality, responses to episodes of ill-health, and choices of treatment (see above). Often the cultures studied have been markedly different from those of the researchers, or have been minority cultures within western societies. On the whole, individuals have been considered to be subsumed within their cultures and have been afforded little autonomy. Lay views of health and illness have consequently been largely disregarded, even by radicals who criticise the power of the medical science monopoly (see Freidson, 1970b, 1973; Illich, 1976; Navarro, 1978; Ehrenreich, 1978; Stoeckle and Barsky, 1981).

"Culture" has also been used within race relations research. It has been adopted in Britain by some writers and politicians to define a "British way of life" which is projected to be a "natural" feeling of the majority white population, and is associated with respectability, thrift, discipline and decency (Hall et al, 1978). Other cultures are then defined as "alien" and "unwanted" (Lawrence, 1982a).

Enoch Powell helped to develop the popular cultural theory of race. He claimed to be speaking with the voice of the majority against the decline of "the English way of life". In the late 1960s, when the recession was just beginning, a panic developed in the media to match Powell's pronouncements, only specifically about a rise in crime rates, particularly those labelled "mugging". There is, in fact, no such crime as mugging, and as Hall (1978; et al, 1978) has shown, it was a phrase borrowed from America to blame street crime on the so-called "enemy within" - the blacks. Hall sees the theory as a development against black people in general, and an ideology created in response to a crisis in economic and political terms - the recession (Hall et al, 1978).

The ideology is based on a desire to return to an idealised version of the past, to a sort of Victorian era of supposed morality, free of crime and controlled by self-discipline - a time that has clearly never existed, but which is attractive to many. The British are assumed in this ideology to be a distinct race, held together by a common culture, a common set of values and beliefs. The next step is to say that it is "natural", therefore, for some people to be prejudiced against outsiders who have a different sort of culture or way of life. The conception of "difference" has arisen from general objections to the imperial and National Front theories of the supposed inferiority of the black race. It is not that blacks are considered inferior, but that they are <u>different</u> (Barker, 1981). This links with the discussion of race in chapter one.

Enoch Powell used the idea of difference to declare that it was only "human nature" to form bounded communities, distinct from others. Thus he promulgated the idea that Britain is the "natural" home of the British; that other people have their own "natural" homes; and that stopping immigration is, therefore, good for immigrants too, because they belong elsewhere (Barker, 1981). When the theory is challenged, it is defended by a form of Darwinist biology which considers that groups are naturally aggressive and competitive, and hostile to "outsiders". The followers of the theory actively deny the superiority theories of the National Front, abhor the suggestion that they might be racists, and claim to be talking "common sense". Thus racism becomes naturalised, and appears to be reasonable, neutral and scientific (Barker, 1981).

References to a British culture or way of life were made in the run-up to the 1979 general election, when Margaret Thatcher declared:

> "If we went on as we are now, then by the end of the century, there would be four million people of the New Commonwealth or Pakistan here. Now that is an awful lot and I think it means that people are really rather afraid that this country might be swamped by people with a different culture. And, you know, the British character has done so much for democracy, for law, and done so much throughout the world, that if there is a fear that it might be swamped, people are going to react, and be rather hostile to those coming in" (Daily Mail, 1978).

These opinions are further expressed and refined in an article by Alfred Sherman, a chief ideologue in the Conservative party, about immigrant workers:

> "There are advantages to employers ... in this flexible supply of cheap, willing labour, outside protective or restrictive legislation and even National Insurance. The costs are borne in the longer term by the nation as a whole. It is not simply the loss to the revenue and National Insurance, but the severe social problems generated by concentrations of people from backward countries, many of whom have little English, who will eventually age, some of whom will give birth to children, often in one parent families, who in turn, given our social arrangements, will be likely to gravitate to the bottom of the social pile " (Guardian, 1984, emphasis added).

It is this use of culture that has been heavily criticised by radical and particularly black writers. They (eg Hall, 1978; CCCS, 1982) have also attacked researchers such as Ballard, Khan (in her early work), and Rapoport, who emphasise that cultural factors are the cause of the disadvantage shown in research by Smith, (1977); Runnymede Trust, (1980); Brown, (1984). The culturalists claim that it is a misunderstanding of and insensitivity to black people's cultures that has resulted in unintentional racial discrimination, and that investigating their culture and educating service providers will eliminate any problems. In education, this is reflected in the DES's policy of multi-cultural education - the aim of which is to teach children about different cultures on equal terms.

There are several flaws in the research which concentrates on culture to the exclusion of all else. Multi-culturalism, and cultural studies in general, tend to assume that cultures are equal in power. In Britain, however, it is clear that cultures are not equally powerful because, for example, most positions of authority, wealth and prestige are held by one small, dominant segment of society: white, middle- and upper-class men. It is the ideology of this group which permeates society and tends to define black people and their families as deviant and problematic (see chapter one; CCCS, 1982). Cultural studies largely ignore the importance of racism, which is, in part, an expression of the unequal power in society.

A concentration on culture is also an "easy" option for policy-makers. Such a concentration focuses attention on individuals and their habits or practices, often emphasising the negative aspects and ignoring the positive effects of culture. Solutions to the "problems" caused by cultural beliefs and practices can then be couched in terms of individual action, by attempting to change people's ways of life rather than trying to understand them. The aim is thus to change the people to match existing services, rather than altering services to meet people's perceived needs.

In the field of health, however, it is neither possible nor desirable to dispense with the concept of culture altogether. It has been shown above that culture defines and selects what sort of ill-health will be perceived, and systematically affects behaviour. It may be, however, that in many cases, social and economic forces (such as the pressure of work, or obligations to friends and relatives) may overcome cultural prescriptions, depending upon their relative powers and the contexts in which they occur. It is postulated in this thesis that the health of black people in Britain depends particularly upon contemporary and historical social, economic and political forces, but that the effects of these forces may be partially eased by behaviour which is inspired by cultural ideas and beliefs. Thus non-white culture should not always be seen in negative terms - it has many positive effects, as the empirical work in this thesis shows.

The use of "culture" as a tool for blaming black people within popular ideology and in research cannot be underestimated. Opposition to this use of culture is also very strong. Although both "race" and "cultural" approaches have some important elements, there have been few studies that draw on both fields. In the general area of the health of black people, the overwhelming majority of research has concentrated on the blaming of individuals and their culture for their ill-health, and there have been only very few studies which have drawn on the literature concerning racial discrimination in the health services and society as a whole. It is the work specifically concerned with "ethnicity" and health that is considered in chapter three.

3 Ethnicity and health

Introduction

This chapter, based largely on Donovan (1982, 1984), is concerned with a review of research which has concentrated on specific diseases and illnesses which are thought to affect black immigrants or their descendants. An analysis of this research on ethnicity and health reveals considerable confusion over the definition of the population that is "ethnic". Words and phrases such as "immigrants", "ethnic minorities", "non-whites", "Asians" and so on tend to be used interchangeably and indiscriminately, often without adequate explanation or definition. The label "immigrant", for example, should refer only to people who have recently entered this country having been born outside the UK, yet it is often used to describe any people who are not white. The use of the word "immigrant" is increasingly inappropriate as the majority of non-whites are born in Britain; and it is also pejorative in tone, suggestive of alien or outsider. Even in its strict sense, the term "immigrant" refers to a highly diverse population, by no means all of whom are of so-called "New Commonwealth" origin.

Evidence about the health status of Britain's black population is patchy and scarce. Even the Black Report, Inequalities and Health, (DHSS, 1980a; Townsend and Davidson, 1982), supposedly the most thorough examination of health in Britain to date, devoted only two or three pages to the health of black Britons (pp58-60, 1982), concentrating instead upon inequalities in health according to class, place of residence, age and gender. A great deal of the research undertaken in the field of ethnicity and health has come from members of the medical profession, published in journals such as the Lancet, British Medical Journal, and Proceedings of the Royal Society of Medicine, and there has been very little contribution from the black population itself or black scholars. Consequently, there has been a bias in the work, characterised by a concentration on illnesses and diseases that interest doctors, central government and the health service administrators:

rickets, tuberculosis and sickle-cell anaemia being examples. This concentration on "interesting" or "unusual" ailments has meant that the assessments and opinions of black people concerning their own health have been largely ignored, as have the obvious links between health and the large and growing literature on "race relations", including levels of deprivation and racial discrimination experienced by black people in Britain. The aim of this chapter is to document this concentration of effort on particular topics and groups at the expense of others. It has been organised in five sections, each of which contains a particular focus of research attention.

Rickets

The re-emergence of the conditions rickets and osteomalacia among children, adolescents and pregnant women of Asian descent living in inner city areas has provoked much emotion as well as research. Most researchers have agreed that, "It seems that vitamin D deficiency is the major factor leading to rickets and osteomalacia among Indian and Pakistani immigrants to Britain" (Preece et al, 1973); but they disagree over precise causes of the affliction and over particular solutions. A large proportion of the research on this disease has been concerned with investigating the number of cases, and discussing possible policy options. In the majority of papers, it is the individual's behaviour, or her/his culture which is blamed, and so solutions are often couched in terms of individual actions with the authorities adopting a "wait and see" approach.

In considering the numbers of cases and who is involved, rickets is seen to have re-appeared among four sections of the Asian population: newborn babies, children, adolescents and pregnant women. Neo-natal rickets, for example, has been found in the babies of Asian women suffering from osteomalacia (Ford et al, 1973), with the babies suffering from softened bones and hypocalcaemic convulsions having acquired the condition "in utero". Ford et al (ibid) alert us to the possibility that, left undetected and/or untreated ante- and post-natally, congenital rickets could become increasingly common. It has been found that giving vitamin D supplements before and after birth will significantly increase the babies' lengths and weights after three months (Brooks, 1981).

Rickets in children has received particular attention. In Birmingham, 51 cases of serious vitamin D deficiency were discovered by Cooke et al (1974) among 31 boys (two of Afro-Caribbean, one of Caucasian, 28 of Asian origin), and 20 girls (three Caucasian, 17 Asian). Between 1968 and 1970, it was reported that 21 Pakistani and Indian children were admitted to Glasgow hospitals with rickets: ten infantile and eleven late; and in the same study, it was shown that of 26 Asian families, 24 per cent suffered from a vitamin D deficiency, and that 20 individuals had biochemical and six radiological evidence of rickets (Ford et al, 1972a). Whether or not such evidence has physiological consequences is not discussed. A large-scale study of 200 Asian, 100 African, 100 Chinese and 100 Scottish children in 1974 revealed that among those of Asian descent, 10 suffered from florid and 15 from sub-clinical rickets, while among the rest there were only seven cases of sub-clinical rickets (three African, three Chinese, one Scot) (Goel et al, 1976). This study was followed up after supplements were given, and in 1979, no children had florid rickets, but nine Asian children still had the sub-clinical form of the disease (Goel et al, 1981).

Adolescents were also found to be badly affected by rickets and osteomalacia. Up to 30 per cent of Asian adolescents and 25 per cent of pregnant women are thought to suffer from mild to severe rickets or osteomalacia (Health and Social Services Journal, 1978). Most of the severe cases were found in adolescents complaining of painful legs (Ford et al, 1972a). In Birmingham, eight men and seventeen women of Asian descent between the ages of eleven and 36 years were admitted to hospital between 1964 and 1970 complaining of limb pain (14), back pain (six), limp (three), fracture (one) and weakness (one) (Swan and Cooke, 1971). The eight men showed a mean average age of 17.6 years, while the women showed two peak ages: pubertal, at 13.8 years, and adult post-pregnancy at 28 years. In most papers, supplements are usually seen as the short-term answer to the condition among adolescents, although Swan and Cooke (ibid) also claim that lack of sunlight may be responsible for the preponderance of women sufferers who were assumed to spend most of their time in the home.

Lack of sunshine is only one of a number of possible causes of rickets. Although researchers agree that a lack of vitamin D is the primary immediate cause of the complaint, this deficiency itself may be caused by any one or a combination of the following: dietary deficiencies, lack of sunshine, the misuse or lack of adequate supplements, and the inhibition of the vitamin by phytate in chapattis - a popular Asian food made from wholemeal flour. Different authors emphasise the importance of different causes, depending on the evidence they have accumulated, but most stay within these four alternatives, although the occasional writer mentions the social and environmental conditions as possible contributors.

Dietary deficiences, for example, are blamed by many for the condition. It seems that Asians fail to eat foods rich in vitamin D, such as oily fish, because of religious restrictions on these foods (BMJ, 1978); or because they are ignorant of foods rich in vitamin D, such as fortified margarine (Smith, 1968); or simply because they choose to eat foods other than those rich in the vitamin, such as ghee (clarified butter) rather than margarine for frying food (Brent CHC, 1981). For some, the answer is simple - "the long term answer to Asian rickets probably lies in health education and a change towards the Western diet and life-style" (Goel et al, 1981, 405), even though these same authors previously admitted that, "one cannot easily change adult dietary habits" (Goel et al, 1976). Such a solution may also be countered by the evidence that the Asian diet is essentially healthy, being near to the WHO ideal, and resulting in much lower rates of heart disease and circulatory problems than does the average Western diet. It may also be added that rickets was largely eradicated among white Britons only when margarine was fortified and milk was given free to children in schools (Brent CHC, 1981). There have been calls for a similar fortification of a popular Asian food (Ford et al, 1972a and b; BMJ, 1979; Arneil and Crosbie, 1963).

One food thought to be suitable for vitamin D fortification is chapatti flour. This is used by large numbers of British Asians - up to 95 per cent are thought to eat chapattis at some time during the week according to Sheiham and Quick, (1982). Although the calls for the fortification of chapatti flour have come from medical experts as well as from the Asian population, the DHSS has refused to sanction it (DHSS,

1980b). The DHSS fears that such fortification might lead to vitamin D overdoses in adults who consume large quantities of chapattis, although the bulkiness of the food would seem to offset this possibility (Sheiham and Quick, 1982). The Department also points out that the amount of chapatti flour consumed varies inversely to the age-group most at risk of rickets, and so supplements may still be required by babies and young children.

There have been suggestions that the high levels of phytate in high fibre foods such as chapatti flour may impair the absorption of vitamin D in the body, and thus increase the likelihood of the incidence of rickets among Asians (Pietrek et al, 1976). Ford et al (1972b) advocate a chapatti-free diet, and claim beneficial results on vitamin D levels when this was enforced among a small group of Asians. It cannot be expected, however, that many Asians will want to give up chapattis entirely and in any case, the evidence about the influence of phytate is not conclusive. It may be that even if phytate does impair the absorption of vitamin D, the fortification of chapatti flour could act to compensate for this (Sheiham and Quick, 1982). At the time of its report, however, the DHSS was unwilling to impose compulsory fortification (even though it still does so in the case of margarine), preferring instead to encourage British Asians to change their diets, use supplements, and expose themselves to more sunlight (DHSS, 1980b).

In the 1980s, the theory that exposure to sunlight is the most important determinant of levels of vitamin D in the blood has taken precedence (Sheiham and Cooke, 1982). A lack of sunshine may be implicated in causing a deficiency of vitamin D because the action of ultra-violet light on the skin stimulates the production of a large part of the body's needs for vitamin D. Arneil and Crosbie (1963), for example, suggest that, "dusky skin requires more ultra-violet radiation than white skin", so black people are supposed to be at a disadvantage in the colder British climate, but the authors fail to explain why people from Africa and the Caribbean do not suffer such high rates of rickets as those of Asian descent. Other authors blame the Asian, and particularly the Muslim, culture which may prevent women from exposing their skin to sunlight (Swan and Cooke, 1971). Again this explanation is unsatisfactory because not all women who practise the Muslim culture strictly suffer from a deficiency of vitamin D, and not all sufferers from rickets are Muslim women. The majority of sufferers live in poor housing in inner city areas. Social conditions, including housing, the local environment, conditions of work, discrimination and poverty are rarely considered as primary causes of rickets and their importance has been underestimated (Brent CHC, 1981).

As a short term solution to rickets, the medical profession and the DHSS are relying upon vitamin supplements which are supposed to be freely available. This is seen, however, as an easy way out - it enables the condition to be treated without offending any individuals or their cultures and is relatively cheap to operate, but it does not do anything to prevent the actual occurrence of the condition and relies upon sufferers to present themselves at the services. The quantities of supplements to treat rickets vary enormously. This is in part a reflection of the various definitions of rickets and deliniations of harmful levels of vitamin D. At present, the most popular test used registers the amount of vitamin D in the blood, but this level does not necessarily correspond with the amount of the vitamin that will be physiologically active, and there seems to be no agreement as to the level that should determine deficiency (Sheiham and Quick, 1982).

Recommendations of treatment for rickets and vitamin D deficiency vary in amount from one high annual dose of vitamin D in the autumn for all children (Stephens et al, 1981), to small amounts of calciferol therapy for twelve months (Cooke et al, 1974). The physiological consequences of rickets are fairly easy to treat amongst babies and children whose bones are still growing, but among adolescents, young women and the elderly, knock-knees, bowed legs, frequent fractures and pelvic deformities may be permanent results, and corrective surgery may be required (Sheiham and Quick, 1982).

The DHSS policy of continuing to use supplements and advocating that Asians should spend more time out of doors and change their diets has been heavily criticised because it is insensitive and ethnocentric. It assumes, for example, that Western diets are healthier than Asian diets, and it gives the impression that Asian diets are to blame for rickets. Similarly, it ignores religious prohibitions on exposing the skin to sunlight, and fails to consider that most sufferers live in crowded inner city areas where there may be few parks and gardens, and where fear of racial attacks may confine people to their homes. There is no evidence to suggest that Asians have a genetic predilection for rickets, and so the primary reasons for its incidence seem likely to be social and environmental, just as they were for the white poor at the turn of the century.

Tuberculosis

The incidence of tuberculosis in immigrants has attracted the attention of many research workers, especially in so far as the disease might pose a threat to the rest of the community (Galloway, 1965). The detection of tuberculosis during medical examinations on entry to Britain was sufficient grounds to deport an individual, or at least to isolate her/him until it could be proved that the disease was no longer infectious. Some studies have attempted to look objectively at the number of cases of tuberculosis recorded in particular groups of immigrants and to suggest possible policy options; others have written more emotively of the risks of letting active sufferers into British cities (Springett et al, 1964).

In general, it appears that rates of tuberculosis are considerably higher among immigrant groups than the indigenous population, although this is not always a result of individuals bringing in the disease themselves (Dodge, 1971). A survey of 843 tuberculosis sufferers (353 of Indian origin, 320 of Pakistani origin, 154 of African origin, and 16 others) showed that only 62 (seven per cent) were found to have the active form of the disease on entry (Khogali, 1979) - strong evidence to support the theory that the majority acquired the disease in the poor and overcrowded housing conditions in Britain's inner cities (Thomas, 1968).

The rates for the notification of tuberculosis in Britain were about 8,000 per annum in the late 1970s (Khogali, 1979) reduced from more than 11,000 cases in 1969, and more than 28,000 in 1959 (Runnymede Trust, 1980). Most of the new cases occur in the newly arrived immigrants, and amongst those who experience very low rates of the disease in their countries of previous residence. The rates for the indigenous population are now very low, at about 0.67 per 1,000 for men, and 0.42 per 1,000 for women (Br. J. Prev. and Soc. Med., 1979), but rates for immigrants are much higher: ten times these figures for Africans, 27 times for Indians, and 54 times for Pakistanis (Khogali, 1979); two times higher for Scots and Europeans, three times higher for Irish, four times higher for West Indians (Springett et al, 1964); and up to 70 times higher for Asians in Leicester (Clarke et al, 1979).

In Britain in 1971, people of recent immigrant origin accounted for less than five per cent of the population, but for 32 per cent of the tuberculosis notifications, with Asians accounting for more than ten per cent of these (Jt. TB Committee, 1978). At a smaller scale, the issue becomes more obvious: among a sample of 2611 catering workers in Soho, 86 had radiological evidence of the disease in the past, 21 had active tuberculosis - an active rate of about eight per 100 sampled, and a rate of 54 per 1,000 among immigrants from Hong Kong (Emerson and Beath, 1961).

Tuberculosis causes about 1,000 deaths per annum in Britain (Clarke et al, 1979), and its treatment costs about forty million pounds per annum (Khogali, 1979), yet very little has been done to curtail its spread. X-rays on entry have been shown to be largely ineffective in detecting other than active cases (Jt. TB Committee, 1978), and calls for vaccination on entry (Springett et al, 1958) would not prevent the spread of the disease among settled immigrants or their friends and families. It is particularly alarming that some immigrants, such as those from the West Indies, came to Britain having little or no experience of tuberculosis in the countries they left, and have acquired the disease here. As far as solutions are concerned, most published papers eventually reach the same conclusion: that it is the environment in the inner cities and the disadvantages experienced by black people that have helped to maintain tuberculosis among them, and that only if and when these conditions are improved, particularly through the provision of adequate, decent housing, will tuberculosis be controlled and reduced (Khogali, 1979).

Inherited Diseases

Inherited diseases usually affect particular sub-groups of the population and have been found among members of ethnic minority groups in

Britain. In particular, genetic diseases such as sickle-cell anaemia and thalassaemia have been found to affect quite substantial proportions of particular groups. Sickle-cell anaemia tends to occur mainly among people of African or Caribbean descent, and has been shown to be quite widely spread in Britain with some concentrations in cities such as London and Birmingham (Davis et al, 1981). Thalassaemia affects a smaller group - principally Greek and Turkish Cypriots, Greeks, Turks, Indians, Pakistanis, some Mediterranean and British people (Thalassaemia Society, 1981). Both diseases exist in two forms: active, where it is extremely painful and can be life-threatening; and passive, where the trait is passed on for generations with no illness present.

Sickle-cell anaemia first occurred in Britain when immigrants arrived from Africa and the Caribbean, where the disease had developed to give partial immunity to endemic malaria (Smith, 1968). The trait of the disease may be found in as many as one in ten babies of Afro-Caribbean descent, but none of these will experience any illness. When two trait carriers plan to have children, however, there is a one in four chance that each baby they have will suffer from sickle-cell anaemia - the life-threatening condition; and a one in two chance that each will carry the trait (Sickle-Cell Society, 1981). Statements of the numbers of sufferers vary: the Sickle-Cell Society estimates that about one in 300 to 400 babies of Afro-Caribbean descent are born with the disease, so they suggest a minimum figure of some 3,000 cases in Britain; a small-scale study by Davis et al (1981) suggests a minimum figure of 1,367 reported cases in Britain; and a recent article puts the figure at at least 4,000, and this is said to be, "the tip of a colossal iceberg", (Konotey-Ahulu, 1982).

The disease has serious implications for the sufferer because it causes red blood cells to become rigid and take on a half-moon shape, and these may then block blood vessels or create clots. This "sickling" may occur after exercise, alcohol, stress, a change in temperature or during pregnancy, and will usually result in extremely painful episodes known as crises in the bones, stomach, back or chest (Sickle-Cell Society, 1981). Complications may include leg ulcers, retarded physical and sexual development (Sarjeant, 1974), stroke, priapism, splenetic infarction and reduced immune response (Sickle-Cell Society, 1981). Infections are often the cause of sudden death at all ages (BMJ, 1975), and patients are particularly susceptible to meningitis, pneumonia and septicaemia (Anionwu and Beattie, 1981).

The health services have been slow in their response to this serious disease. There is only one Sickle-Cell Centre in Britain, at Willesden Hospital, London, and surveys have shown that many doctors and medical professionals are not aware of the symptoms and dangers of the disease and so may not always recognise it (Sickle-Cell Society, 1981). A survey of 227 haematologists in 197 centres all over Britain revealed 1367 reported cases of sickle-cell anaemia in 1978-9; that there were sickle-cell clinics at only 13 per cent of these centres; that only two-thirds of the centres examined "at risk" pregnant women ante-natally; and that only one-third of the centres screened new-born babies for the trait or the disease (Davis et al, 1981).

Treatment of the condition has been inadequate, and although bone marrow transplants and genetic surgery may be possible in the future (Lehmann, 1974), at present treatment is merely an attempt to alleviate the pain suffered during crises, by pain killing drugs and increasing fluid intake (Anionwu and Beattie, 1981). The survey by Davis et al (1981) showed that folic acid was given at only 80 per cent of centres, penicillin at only 24 per cent, and vaccine for menengitis at only four out of 197 centres - yet the last two are essential to prevent infections after crises. Life expectancy for a sufferer is reasonable once adulthood is reached, but nearly 50 per cent of deaths occur at or under six years of age (Davis et al, ibid).

Thalassaemia has a slightly different pattern and affects people of different ethnic origins. Thalassaemia-minor (carrying the trait), has no ill-effects, but involves about one in seven Cypriots, one in twelve Greeks, one in twenty Turks, Indians and Pakistanis, and one in 1,000 British (Thalassaemia Society, 1981). Again, the trait has little importance until two carriers have children, when there is a one in four chance of each child having thalassaemia-major. This takes two forms: one which is fatal before or soon after birth, and another in which the baby is apparently healthy at birth, but becomes ill later. Unlike sickle-cell anaemia sufferers, those with thalassaemia-major require transfusions of blood every four to six weeks, otherwise they may die (Modele et al, 1980). Life expectancy is low because of the complications of iron-poisoning, liver and spleen diseases, heart failure and diabetes (Thalassaemia Society, 1981). Even if children survive, they may suffer retarded growth, delayed puberty and skin pigmentation (Knox-Macaulay et al, 1973). There are thought to be about 300 thalassaemia-major sufferers in Britain, two-thirds of whom are of Cypriot origin (Modele et al, 1980). The risk for Cypriots is particularly high: a Cypriot woman carrying thalassaemia trait has a one in 28 chance of having a thalassaemia-major child: 15 such children are born in Britain each year.

The number of sufferers of both thalassaemia and sickle-cell anaemia seems likely to increase in the near future as the black population increases. The Sickle-Cell Society (1981) has called for better training of health professionals, the dissemination of information to the community, special allocation of funds to study the disease, better housing and education facilities for sufferers, and, in particular, exemption from prescription charges for all those suffering from inherited diseases such as sickle-cell anaemia. It has also demanded routine screening on request for all "at risk", especially babies, pregnant women and those about to have operations, but it contends that such screening must be accompanied by sufficient numbers of trained counsellors. It is now possible to detect whether or not a foetus has the disease by amniocentesis (Times, 1981), but attempts to encourage the abortion of these foetuses without adequate counselling have been met with allegations of genocide (Konotey-Ahulu, 1982). As yet, most of the information about sickle-cell anaemia and thalassaemia has come from "ad hoc" societies run as charities, and the NHS and DHSS seem happy to let this continue. The DHSS is apparently considering whether or not to allocate some funds to the Sickle-Cell Society, but it has not yet formulated any clear policy on either disease.

Mental Health

Turning from the research into the physical health of black people, it is essential to consider the literature on mental health and ethnicity. The evidence from much of this work is, however, somewhat contradictory. Psychology and psychiatry have been criticised for past involvement in the justification of imperialism and slavery (Sashidharan,

1981), and in deeming some ethnic groups inferior so that they might be dominated or even exterminated - as happened to the Jews in Nazi Germany. More recently, psychology and psychiatry have been concerned with explaining migrant behaviour and the effects of migration on the mental health of the individual and/or group. On the whole, it is suggested that moving from a poor rural area in a Third World country to a large British city is a stressful experience, and that when this is compounded by "culture shock" and racial discrimination, high rates of mental illness are only to be expected (CRC, 1976; BMJ, 1980; Rack, 1979). Poverty and downward occupational and social mobility have also been suggested as factors causing high rates of mental instability (MIND, 1976). Among Asians, it is claimed, these problems are further compounded by language difficulties, and for the women especially, isolation without the traditional extended family (Schofield, 1981). For West Indians, frustration at not being accepted by British society, and difficulties with children who reject their colour and ethnic background, are seen as extra causes of anxiety (CRC, 1976; Hashmi, 1970).

The contradiction arises, however, when one looks at studies of actual use of psychiatric services or figures for attendance at mental institutions, where it appears that black people do not use psychiatric services as much as white people do. Asians, for example, show much lower rates of disturbance and admittance to mental hospitals than either white people or other immigrants (Cochrane, 1979a); and much lower suicide rates than other groups (Burke, 1976). The picture for those of West Indian origin is somewhat different: although their rates for affective and depressive illnesses are markedly lower than for the majority of the population (Hitch, 1981), their rates for schizophrenia, and for children's attendance at schools for the educationally sub-normal, are much higher than in other groups (Gordon, 1965; Cochrane, 1979b; Klein, 1979).

Explanations for these apparent contradictions vary. Those who maintain that high rates of instability should be expected explain the figures which show low rates of utilizing services as indicative of a failure of the services themselves; or by suggesting that the stigma of insanity is so great that a large proportion of real illness is concealed by the families of the sufferers; or by indicating that perhaps the ethnic groups themselves provide sufficient non-professional treatment to prevent the mentally ill from turning to the authorities (Rack, 1979; MIND, 1976). Other researchers invoke cultural factors which, they maintain, explain and contain mental illness in ethnic groups (Kiev, 1964; Runnymede Trust, 1980). Cochrane and Stopes-Roe (1980) postulate that there is no necessary association between migration and vulnerability to mental illness. Emphasis is placed in a few papers on a consideration of the differences in the reporting of symptoms by people of different cultures to their British general practitioners, and there have been calls for much greater consideration of methods of symptom presentation because they are so crucial to a correct diagnosis of mental illness (Rack in Runnymede Trust, 1980; Littlewood and Lipsedge, 1982).

Psychiatrists and doctors in general need to be aware of, and sensitive to, their patients' cultures if they are not to misunderstand the behaviour presented to them. Studies have been undertaken to look at cultural responses to, for example, depression, and it does appear that different groups may have different ways of expressing this ailment based on their cultural perceptions of it. Asians, when attending psychiatric services (which is rare), seem to focus their attention on physical complaints such as sexual impotence if they are male (Hashmi, 1966), or on sleeplessness, sweating, headaches, and "spinning head" if female (Ingham, 1981); whereas West Indians tend to concentrate on the loss of strength and inability to work if male (Hashmi, 1966), or on fertility and headaches if female (Carne, 1970). These summaries of symptoms are obviously over-generalised and very limited, but they do illustrate the possibility of an inadequately trained or insensitive doctor making a serious diagnostic error.

Such errors have been suggested to occur in the diagnosis of schizophrenia and deviance among black, and particularly West Indian adults and children (BMJ, 1980). In a Bradford hospital study, it was found that immigrants from the New Commonwealth were diagnosed with far more schizophrenia and paranoia, and far fewer affective and depressive illnesses, than white British patients (Hitch, 1981). Similarly, in Nottingham over seven years, 29 per cent of schizophrenic notifications were of members of ethnic minorities, even though they accounted for only 6.5 per cent of the city's population (Alexander, 1974). Finally, a study in an east London hospital showed that about 41 per cent of West Indian patients were diagnosed with schizophrenia, compared with only 20 per cent of white patients (Gordon, 1965). The tendency for black patients to be more readily diagnosed as schizophrenic than white patients may be caused by doctors failing to understand acceptable behaviour: a survey of 100 youths of West Indian origin revealed that almost all experienced religious or magical delusions and did not believe this to be abnormal or unusual (Kiev, 1964).

A final example of work in this field provides some evidence of racism among members of staff in their diagnosis and treatment of black patients. The study involved an analysis of outpatients to an east London District General Hospital, and a closer look at those patients who had received electro-convulsive therapy (ECT) over 18 months (Littlewood and Cross, 1980). Among the outpatients, it became evident that blacks were much more likely than their white counterparts to receive physical treatments, especially major tranquilizers and ECT; to receive intra-muscular medication, and to have an outpatient attendance pattern involving self-referral, missed appointments and being seen only by junior, often black, members of staff. Among those receiving ECT, black patients appeared to be perceived by staff as in greater need of this therapy than other groups - even though they were rarely diagnosed as depressed. The authors suggest that these evident misdiagnoses appear to involve either differences in psychiatric phenomenology not yet recognised by the profession as a whole, or in the stereotyped attitudes and racism of mental health professionals (Littlewood and Cross, 1980).

Some workers have looked in detail at the ways in which mental illnesses are diagnosed, and have shown that cultural perceptions are of the utmost importance in defining normality and deviance, on which such diagnoses are based. It may be, therefore, that behaviour in Britain not following the cliched "stiff upper lip" tradition, for example, may be diagnosed as schizophrenic here, although acceptable in another country or culture. Littlewood and Lipsedge, (1982), have also suggested that an episode of schizophrenia or paranoia in a black person may be an understandable reaction to the institutionalised and personal racism which she/he faces in Britain. It may be that racism, in society and psychiatry, will prove to be the major cause of differences in rates of mental illness between ethnic groups. The re-appraisal and reform of the treatment of mental illness in black people, so urgently required, must take this into account.

Health and the Family

There has been some interest in the field of ethnicity and health in the "family", and particularly how cultural differences in family composition might affect health. Studies of people of Asian descent have tended to concentrate on the issues of infant and peri-natal mortality, low birthweights, and the difficulties thought to be suffered by women who may not have the support of a traditional extended family in Britain. The studies of people of Afro-Caribbean descent, however, have had quite different foci: researchers have been much more concerned with the effects on children's health of one-parent families and mothers who work and raise children concurrently.

Researchers have shown concern about the discovery of high infant mortality figures among Asians, even when the women involved are put in a "low risk" category by virtue of their age and parity (Terry et al, 1980). It has been suggested that the high infant mortality rates of 15.1 per 1,000 for still births, and 27.5 per 1,000 for peri-natal deaths can be explained by the small stature of Asian women, nutritional deficiencies, anaemia, short pregnancy intervals, or their concentration in the lowest social classes with the poorest housing and lowest incomes (Lumb et al, 1981). In data from the Bradford Health Authority, the apparent high rates of Asian peri-natal mortality are not significant if the class position of mothers is taken into account (Pearson, 1983). Similarly, in data collected by the OPCS for the GLC, it has been shown that the high peri-natal and infant mortality rates among Asians are paralleled in social classes IV and V, and since the majority of Asians fall into these classes, ethnic differences may again not be significant (GLC, 1982).

There has also been publicity about the so-called "problems" of low birthweights and slow physical development of Asian babies, yet such "evidence" as has been produced is usually based on height and weight charts designed for the average white middle-class baby, without adjustments for the smaller average stature of Asian mothers, their gynaecological history, or their class position in Britain. One survey done some time ago of 6,000 infants in a Lambeth hospital showed that differences in birthweight means could not be explained exclusively by nationality, social class, maternal health and welfare, or the duration of gestation (Barron and Vessey, 1966). This survey highlights the fact that there have so far been inadequate and partial investigations of the issues of low birthweights, low rates of utilization of ante- and post-natal services, and high infant and perinatal mortality rates.

Studies of the "family" usually invoke the "typical" British pattern of two adults (married) and one or two children as the norm or ideal, and sometimes fail to appreciate the disadvantage of this and/or the advantages of some other family structures to some people. Research into factors affecting the health of the families of Afro-Caribbean origin, for example, has been interested in the central role of the mother, and her difficulties in working and rearing children simultaneously in poor environmental conditions. Some nutritional disorders appear to arise in babies kept on milk alone until the age of two years (Gans, 1966) and high rates of accidental injury have been reported among children of West Indian origin (Patterson, 1966).

A study of West Indian one year olds in Paddington showed that their mothers used the health services as much as white mothers, that they tended to have more treatment for minor ailments and to be admitted to hospital more often than the white group, that their mothers tended to work and leave them with child-minders (70 per cent of whom were not registered), and, most important, that housing conditions were poor and that most of the illnesses suffered - anaemia, eczema, upper and lower respiratory tract infections - were explicable with reference to overcrowded housing with few toilets, poor washing facilities and limited heating (Pless and Hood, 1967). Also mentioned has been the extra problem of racial discrimination and possible differences in the quality of treatment received by black people (Oppe, 1964; Pless and Hood, 1967).

Some authors have considered the effects on health of the large number of one-parent families (13 per cent of West Indian compared with nine per cent of the rest of the population), and the numbers of mothers employed outside the home. These factors have been implicated in the higher incidence of burn accidents in West Indian homes (Patterson, 1964), although the reliance on cheap but dangerous paraffin heaters is a more likely cause of this; or in the over-representation of black children in care (48 per cent in Wandsworth) (Runnymede Trust, 1980), although the lack of official day nursery and child-minding services may also be implicated here.

There have been a small number of studies of the use of traditional medicines and healers by members of ethnic groups in Britain. Most of the research has concerned the use of hakims, practitioners of the Unani school of medicine based in southern Asia, who have been located in Bradford (Davis and Aslam, 1980). These healers treat patients holistically, concentrating on the balance of humours within the body, particularly the forces of hot and cold as they affect ill-health (Davis and Aslam, ibid; Eagle, 1980; Aslam et al, 1981). There are even fewer studies of the use of traditional healing methods among people of Afro-Caribbean descent, even though Kitzinger (1980) discovered that many of the people she talked to had non-scientific conceptions of how the body works, and regularly used some home remedies. It is one of the aims of this thesis to expand upon this limited information.

The health of elderly black people has not been considered until recently because of the large proportion of the black population in the young age groups. The number of elderly (over 65 years) has been estimated at 26,400 (Glendenning, 1980); or 32,000 (Mays, 1981), and this is likely to increase greatly in the near future when the present middle-aged cohort moves into the over 60s age group. A recent estimate suggests that the number of black people over the age of 65 years is likely to rise from about 40,000 now to at least 200,000 by the turn of the century (Brass, 1983). Particular problems of the elderly are common to all ethnic groups: poor housing, low incomes, increased morbidity, limited mobility and so on, but for black people these may be compounded by racial discrimination, loss of a sense of home, language difficulties, isolation, and rejection by the young of their traditional role as respected elders (Glendenning, 1980). They may also face extra difficulties of understanding and being aware of claims for assistance, and so may fail to receive their entitlements to 'bus passes, home-helps and even pensions (Mays, 1981). Extra funds or a shift of resources will soon be necessary if the health and welfare services are to cope with these new demands.

Conclusion

The study of ethnicity and health thus revolves principally around a few major illnesses and diseases that have captured the attention of medical and other professionals, but which affect relatively small numbers of black people. Although these illnesses are important and need treatment, they do not represent the everyday health problems that most black people have to contend with. One piece of work shows this quite clearly: it is an analysis of telephone calls to a London radio station offering guidance on health matters in a variety of languages where callers could talk in confidence to members of their own ethnic groups (Webb, 1981). The majority of callers were Asian men, many requiring information on their wives' behalf, and most calls concerned day to day worries about asthma, psychosexual problems, diabetes, nutrition and mental health. West Indian callers were more interested in information about services rather than health problems. Although the sample is not necessarily representative of the black population, it does show that there are differences between the perceptions of the professionals and of the people over which health problems are of particular importance.

Concentrating interest on specific diseases or illnesses that affect particular ethnic groups has the effect of singling out some groups of people as "problems". The illnesses considered are themselves almost always referred to as "problems", and are often seen to arise from cultural practices. Thus the Asian diet is blamed for rickets and low birthweight babies; and West Indian family patterns are blamed for child accident rates and the numbers of children in care. The placing of blame on the individual or the culture of origin is a commonly used method of social control, and means that the "solutions" to the "problems" may be couched in terms of individual action without involving financial expenditure or changes in social and economic structures. Health education is used in this way, although its attempts to change dietary and family patterns are unlikely to be any more successful than its recent attempts to curtail smoking among people in social classes IV and V. People do not perceive that their traditional diets and family patterns are primary causes of their ill-health - the actions of the state and the class system are much more obviously involved.

Thus the health of black people in Britain today is dependent upon the interplay of culture and race. Culture can have many positive effects, although these have rarely emerged from the studies concerned with ethnicity and health, where culture is usually taken to be problematic. As indicated in chapter two, culture influences health in many ways, particularly through its delimitation of what an illness is, and its "recipes" for dealing with episodes of ill-health. A person's cultural heritage may also provide her/him with a set of tried and tested traditional remedies which have been largely ignored by researchers and the medical profession.

Race is involved through the effects of racism and racial discrimination on the position of black people in contemporary Britain. The Black Report, Inequalities in Health, (DHSS, 1980a), showed the immense importance of the class structure in creating and perpetuating inequalities in the health of white Britons, but it conspicuously failed to go on to examine the health of the black population. "Race relations" research (see chapter one) has shown that the majority of the black population is caught in the lowest social classes, with some of the most dangerous and lowest paid jobs, the worst housing, and living in some of the worst environmental conditions in the inner cities (Rose, 1969; Sivanandan, 1982; Brown, 1984). An additional and extremely important factor is that of racism which has also been well documented in its effects on black people (Smith, 1977; Brown, 1984). These factors can be implicated in all of the illnesses considered above, with the exception of the inherited conditions.

Despite this evidence, the pamphlet by the Brent Community Health Council (1981) is one of very few publications which does attempt to link the health of black people to the social, political and economic constraints within which they live. It is the aim of this thesis to examine the health of black people as they see it, and to set the study within the context of contemporary "race relations".

4 The methodological background

Introduction

This chapter is concerned with the exposition of the methodology of the field research which is reported in the chapters that follow. The methodology draws heavily on the sociological critique of positivism, and the postulations of the interpretative school of sociology. Anthropological work is also considered, particularly that concerning ethnography, analytic induction and the use of the case-study approach. The methodology is essentially eclectic, drawing upon several schools of thought.

The importance of these viewpoints to this study emerged from the critique of much of the research concerning the health of black people in Britain (see chapter three). This research, chiefly undertaken by medical professionals, has tended to follow the methodology of the natural sciences, and has focused attention onto particular topics and ethnic groups at the expense of others (see also Donovan, 1984). Much of this work has used quantitative techniques to measure the incidence of particular conditions within specific groups, and there has been very little qualitative work looking at the experience of health and illness from the point of view of black people.

The neglect of lay perceptions of health and illness was touched upon in chapter two. This neglect is also related to the reliance of much traditional social science on a methodology borrowed from the physical sciences. This thesis aims to break away from this tradition, presenting a qualitative study of black people's perceptions and experiences of health, illness and the health services, which draws more upon the methodology of interpretative sociology and ethnography than on social science modelled on the physical sciences.

INTERPRETATIVE SOCIOLOGY

The interpretative "school" in sociology developed out of the hermeneutic philosophy of the eighteenth century as an alternative to the theories and methods of positivists and structural-functionalists. It draws upon the hermeneutic tradition, with its emphasis on the centrality of "verstehen" (understanding), and the importance of the interpretative understanding of human action (Giddens, 1976). It is not a unified school, but consists of several fairly distinct groups, all critical of natural scientific theories and methods and demanding that the central concern of sociology should be the meanings of the social world, but each proposing different methodological frameworks and theoretical principles. The most obvious groupings are the phenomenologists, the symbolic interactionists, and the ethnomethodologists. Other writers share the phenomenological critique of traditional sociology but are not part of a specific grouping - these include anthropologists, ethnographers and individuals such as Glaser, Strauss and Weber.

Increasing dissatisfaction with the results of sociological work carried out according to the methodology of the natural sciences or some adaptation of this led to the re-examination of the bases of social research. Radicals and others had been questioning the usefulness of the positivistic and scientistic paradigms for some time, and some anthropologists had been developing and refining qualitative techniques. At first, however, the "interpretative sociologists" (as they came to be known) concentrated on a thorough critique of positivism and an expose of the biases hidden by so-called neutral numerical analyses. Some then concentrated on producing theories for sociological work; others on attempts to develop methods for empirical work.

Positivistic methods have been used in sociological work to try to develop social science in the same way as natural science. The failure of positivistic sociology to find convincing scientific explanations for social phenomena have been, subsequently, put down to the unsophisticated nature of the discipline, and methodological problems have been treated as teething troubles of a young science (Walsh, 1972c). The primacy of positivism has been defended, then, by maintaining that social science will always be developing. When the data fail to fit the theory, positivist writers rely on their own common-sense interpretations to explain what is going on, and these may fit the theory but are rarely demonstrated by the evidence. One such example can be seen in Durkheim's study of suicide (1952) where in order for his data to be consistent with the theory, he had to "make up" elaborate and tortuous conceptions of the differences between male and female minds (Douglas, 1971).

Natural science has derived much of its strength from the consensus of scientists and its confidence in its taken-for-granted paradigm (Walsh, 1972a). When scientific methods are applied to the social world, the meanings and values of individuals have to be modelled and the social world has to become akin to the natural world of material facts which is thought to be neutrally observable and part of an established homeostatic system (see Parsons, 1951; Durkheim, 1938, 1960). Only things that are measurable can be considered and the emphasis of the studies is placed on the methods of systematic observation, replication and prediction (Walsh, 1972a). It was assumed that sociology would become a science through the quantitative verification of hypotheses (Glaser and Strauss, 1967), and that universal laws would be discovered which could lead to prediction and, ultimately, social control. These views have been heavily criticised by radicals and followers of the interpretative school of sociology.

Critics have suggested that adopting positivistic methods have led to studies designed only in accordance with "proper form" and without any reference to the subject matter concerned (Louch, 1966). For many, the prevailing social science paradigm is seen to be out of step with reality, resting on assumptions neither acknowledged nor verified (Phillipson, 1972b), and where theory just "arises" with no question of from where it arises (Silverman, 1972b). Others criticise the way in which positivists claim that their methods are neutral: in fact social surveys and scientific practices contain implicit theories and assumptions that are seldom investigated or justified. Similarly, positivistic methods use statistics which are assumed to be rational and neutral tools, without attempts to analyse the biases that may exist (Phillipson, 1972a). Leading on from these criticisms is the question of how measurement is imposed upon the social world and why numbers appear to give respectability and neutrality to studies when they may actually dehumanise the research and are themselves the product of common-sense and intuitive decisions by individual researchers (Phillipson, 1972a).

Some radical writers have also criticised the use of positivistic methodologies in sociological work. There is an essential tension within radical research between the attempts to produce scholarly work and the necessity to criticise the status quo and to effect change. As Colfax (1971) points out, just as empiricism served to keep social scientists away from examining the values implicit in their work, so the need for scholarship has allowed radicals to avoid the dilemma of whether or not to act. The major focus of interest for many radicals has been to analyse the workings and structures of society, and there have been criticisms that the individual is thus overlooked. Some radicals have chosen to direct their criticism towards orthodox social science. Positivism is thus seen to maintain the status quo of corporate capitalism and exploitation, while at the same time asserting its objectivity and neutrality (Colfax and Roach, 1971).

Feminists who have criticised traditional social science consider that the lives of women have been excluded from the majority of studies, or have been portrayed in sexist ways (Roberts, 1981; Graham, 1982; Keohane et al, 1982). This is a consequence of the fact that traditional social theory has been developed largely by men and has built upon men's relation to the social world. Social surveys have also been criticised for obscuring relationships that mould people's lives because they ignore everyday conversations and seek to place experiences in pre-defined categories. Like other radicals, feminists also criticise the ways in which positivistic theories represent the status quo as neutral and benign, thus obscuring the true nature and pattern of power in Western society which is still held largely by white, middle-class men.

In the field of medical sociology, the application of positivistic methods has highlighted the gap between lay and professional views of health and illness. Positivistic sociological theory posits a benign medical profession and system using their neutral, scientific tools and methods to maintain a population healthy enough to carry out its social roles. Lay views of health and illness are seen to be inferior, partial and irrational in comparison with the superior, scientific and rational theories of medicine (Freidson, 1970b). Parsons was a chief exponent of positivistic medical sociology. His work on the Social System (1951), for example, elaborated his ideas on the reciprocal and consensual nature of the doctor-patient relationship, in which the patient, who temporarily adopts the sick role, is obliged to see a physician and to "co-operate with him (sic) in the process of trying to get well" (437). The patient thus defers to the judgement of the physician over matters of health.

Other medical sociologists have studied "illness behaviour" in terms of the individual, rarely challenging or criticising the service providers (see Mechanic, 1978; Zborowsky in Stoeckle and Barsky, 1981). Medicine is thus seen to be correct and unchallengeable. Such a view has been heavily criticised by humanists and radicals such as Illich (1976), Navarro (1978) and Ehrenreich (1978) who see medicine much more in terms of its definition as an institution of social control and its gradual take over of large sections of life (the so-called medicalisation of life). They see the clinical encounter between patient and doctor as being an unequal meeting, comprising conflict rather than consensus, and in which the doctor holds the power. Conflict arises particularly when the physician is of a different class or culture from her/his patients. On the whole, however, radicals still tend to treat the lay population as a unitary whole (which it clearly is not) and they largely consider the lay perceptions of ordinary people to be of little account.

Some radicals, such as Feyerabend (1970), suggest dispensing with method altogether because set methodologies do not allow a sense of history, nor do they enable the researcher to deal with unexpected discoveries. Phillips suggests that, "method is antithetical to the openness of experience" (1973, 164), and he advocates abandoning method. Phillips believes that a strict adherence to a method prevents the researcher from seeing things as they really are, and he points out that methods are the construction of researchers and so should not be accepted uncritically.

Positivism thus has very little to offer a study aiming to uncover the meanings, perceptions and experiences of health and illness. Positivistic methodology offers a well-established and widely accepted but taken-for-granted methodology, but such a methodology is usually imposed without a sensitive concern for the subject matter, and it does not necessarily reflect the experiences of the people under study. Positivistic social surveys can offer tested questionnaires, but they may be ethnocentric and, as Cicourel (1964) points out, interviewers tend to reduce the complexity of respondents' accounts by placing them into arbitrary classification systems based upon the researcher's own implicit assumptions. If one is aiming to explore the complexity of issues, this is clearly not useful. Structural-functional theory, which postulates society as a self-balancing system based on consensus, is also inappropriate for a study looking at an oppressed group in society, whose position can be clearly seen to be the result of conflict and inequality dating from the imperial era to the present (see chapter one; Sivanandan, 1982; Brown, 1984).

The traditional social survey is inappropriate for this project because it fails to allow people freedom to describe and explain their own lives in their own ways. Social surveys are designed to elicit replies in particular ways, and do not allow researchers to alter the wording or order of questions. Social survey questionnaires can force people into opinions they do not really hold (Manning, 1967), and they assume that all people will respond in the same ways and that the meanings of the questions will be the same for all respondents (Denzin, 1978). Social surveys fail to consider the importance of the presentation of the interview, the relationship between the interviewer and the subject, and do not allow for a consideration of the uniqueness of each individual's way of perceiving and defining the world (Denzin, 1978). Social survey instruments may also be ethnocentric since the majority of them are written to elicit the views of the majority white population.

Traditional methods of sampling respondents are also neither appropriate nor necessary for this study. There are many practical difficulties about using random sampling from the usual sources such as electoral registers or rating lists. Firstly, black people tend not to be fully registered on electoral rolls for a variety of reasons including the mobility of people in the inner-city areas in which they tend to live, the lack of information about how to register for those with a limited amount of English, the misunderstanding by registrars of the correct forms of people's names, and a lack of interest in elections where black issues are rarely touched upon. Another difficulty with the use of electoral registers and rating lists is that black people are "invisible": names, for example, are not an accurate representation of people's ethnic origins. Census data are of little use because questions are not asked of people's ethnic and racial identity, and since the majority of black people have now been born in Britain, birthplace data are of little relevance. These restrictions prevent the carrying out of an orthodox, statistically representative social survey.

The aim of the study, to understand health and illness in the context of people's lives, demands, therefore, a methodology that is not taken directly from traditional positivistic research, nor from research undertaken by medical professionals (see chapter three). The study calls for a methodology which is sensitive and flexible, and considers the views and opinions of ordinary people in their own terms. Such a methodology is supported by work in phenomenology, ethnomethodology, symbolic interactionism and ethnography. These are considered in some detail, below.

Phenomenology

Phenomenology is derived largely from the philosophy of Husserl. Husserl believed that all consciousness is intentional and saw the aim of phenomenology to uncover pure subjectivity by clearing away all that is taken for granted (Giddens, 1976). As an early critic of the structural-functionalists, Max Weber played an important role in using some of Husserl's ideas in relation to social studies. Weber was concerned that the individual should be the fundamental unit of investigation, and argued consistently that the individual was much more important than "the system". He also believed that each individual was capable of meaningful social action (Parkin, 1982). Weber saw sociology's aim as getting at the motives for social action by somehow penetrating the subjective understanding of the individual. His method for such investigation was termed "verstehen": to empathise totally with the subject, to identify with her/him. In this process, the researcher should view the subject's actions through her/his eyes and thus discover motives behind the behaviour.

Weber also introduced the concept of "ideal types" to be drawn up by the researcher and against which empirical cases could be compared and evaluated. These ideal types represent an accentuation of the characteristics of cultural values, patterns of actions and events into an abstract "ideal" form (Hirst, 1976). They comprise, therefore, a sort of "model" against which reality can be measured. Weber calls in his work for a value-free social science to be developed, but it is hard to envisage how the methods of verstehen and ideal types can be free from researchers' pre-judgements or biases. The construction of ideal types also ensures that "rational action" remains the norm, and so conventionalism tends to be the outcome (Hirst, 1976). Weber is important to the interpretative school, however, because of his critique of positivism and his insistence on the primacy of a thinking, choosing individual, able to make sense of the world through the attachment of meanings to social phenomena.

The phenomenological critique alleges that methods adopted from the natural sciences miss the "sense" of phenomena by using methods which detach them from their specific contexts (Phillipson, 1972b). The relevance of phenomenology to this study, then, is that it aims to study phenomena in their own terms so that their integrity is not lost (Douglas, 1971); and to seek an understanding of the ways in which people make sense of their lives and the (social) worlds they live in. For specific behaviour such as an individual's response to an illness to be understandable, the phenomenologists claim, the meanings that people attach to their actions and the processes by which people act out their everyday lives must be investigated. Some phenomenologists take as the focus of their study the "taken-for-granted" and common-sense ideas which permeate daily activities (see, for example, Berger and Luckmann, 1966).

Researchers of the interpretative school are interested in how the social world is created and maintained. Unlike the natural world, which has no intrinsic meaning, the social world is inherently meaningful because it is made by people and created and re-created in every social encounter (Giddens, 1976). The processes of this production and reproduction of the social world are crucial to phenomenological enquiry, because these processes are themselves "uniquely meaningful" (Silverman, 1972c). Phenomenological philosophy has as its aim the total understanding of consciousness, but most researchers realise that this is an ideal and not possible because they cannot get inside their subject's heads in order to perceive the world as they perceive it. Hence the concentration on understanding the processes of experience, with the generally accepted assumption that others experience things in a similar way - that "the other knows as I know" (Silverman, 1972b).

The way in which the social world becomes available and constituted is the subject of phenomenological sociology (Walsh, 1972a). Social facts are not seen "as if they were things" (Durkheim's view), but as the practical accomplishment of the routine practices and experiences of people in their ordinary lives. These social facts are sustained and re-affirmed in the course of social interaction (conversations etc). Some of them are commonly held and have the same meanings for groups of people; others have meanings which are negotiated during conversation or experience. The phenomenologists stress the importance of the negotiable nature of the social world and social order (Walsh, 1972c) - an order which is shared by a social group, but always open to challenges and re-negotiation. The individual is thus allowed some choice in her/his life. The phenomenologists, however, largely fail to consider the importance of power in relationships. In the health sphere, for example, lay and professional ideas about health and illness are accorded equivalent status by phenomenologists because they are social constructions, but, in fact, professional ideas are dominant because of their monopoly of knowledge and, therefore, power.

The meanings of social facts, social processes and the social world are other foci of interest for phenomenologists. All human beings are assumed to have consciousness, and this is also assumed to be intentional (Phillipson, 1972b). The intentional nature of consciousness is its ability to assign meanings to things, and since the consciousness is directed toward the "life world" (the world we live in), meanings are given to all things that come to its attention within its horizons. Every individual has a unique stock of knowledge based on previous experiences and inherited ideas, some of which she/he shares with others. Social order is established through the sharing of some meanings, usually in the form of common-sense (Walsh, 1972a; Berger and Luckmann, 1966).

Common-sense is defined by Gramsci to be the uncritical and largely unconscious way in which people perceive the world, and which consists of confused and contradictory ideas composed of folk-lore, myths and popular experiences (Gramsci in Simon, 1982). According to Gramsci, common-sense is not created in every context, but is the outcome of unequal negotiations between the dominant ideology and individuals. It may, therefore, contain elements of the dominant ideology which individuals do not fully share. Schutz (1972), however, contends that an individual's stock of knowledge (which includes common-sense) is constantly revised during interactions with others, depending upon the context. Thus interactions between individuals can lead to the challenging and up-dating of each individual's stock of knowledge (Berger and Kellner, 1970). This does not usually lead to the disturbing or challenging of the status quo, however, because common-sense can contain contradictory ideas. Individual or group perceptions may be altered by new circumstances, therefore, but the status quo remains intact.

Weber's ideas about ideal types have been taken up by other interpretative thinkers such as Schutz (see below). The meanings which people hold in common are taken to be typifications or ideal types of the phenomena. These common-sense understandings are not formal rules, but are the outcome of contemporary interpretations of what is going on in everyday life (Walsh, 1972a). Hence racism, according to this analysis, may be the outcome of conceptions of "ideal" or "stereo" types, in which, typically, whites are seen as superior and blacks inferior in a number of ways. Whether or not this conception of racism as inevitable and inherent in people's consciousness is accurate is contentious, however, and other views of racism have been elaborated elsewhere (see chapters one and two).

It is perhaps germane here to consider the importance of the contribution of Schutz to the phenomenological paradigm. It is probably Schutz more that any other individual who has established phenomenology as an alternative to positivism and structural functionalism in sociology. Schutz claims that his writings draw directly on the philosophy of Husserl, although his critics claim that he has imposed his own ideas on Husserl's, and so his foundations are not truly phenomenological (Hindess, 1972; Gorman, 1975). Of particular importance to this thesis are Schutz's developments of some of the ideas first postulated by Weber, such as the role of consciousness in giving meanings to phenomena, the importance of common-sense interpretations of reality, and the role of ideal types in everyday interaction. Most of these developments are contained in Schutz's major work, The Phenomenology of the Social World, (1972).

Schutz thought that the aim of the social sciences should be to interpret (that is, understand) the subjective meaning of social action. He saw action as defined through meaning. A major development of Schutz's theory was that the stream of consciousness of each individual had no intrinsic meaning, but that once an experience had passed, it would be lifted out of the stream of consciousness to become a distinct entity endowed with meaning. Schutz believed that one had to assume that another person's perceptions were almost identical to one's own, and that the most important social interaction was the face-to-face relationship in which each member is able to perceive the other directly. This is in contrast to the relationship each individual has with her/his predecessors and successors, where knowledge of them is clearly indirect. Schutz postulated that when individuals are interpreting the behaviour of their contemporaries, they use ideal types, and that these ideal types are the fundamental tool of the social sciences.

Although Schutz borrowed Weber's ideas about the importance of individual perceptions and the formulation of ideal types, he thought the social world was much more complex than Weber did. Schutz believed that the social world was a complex system of perceptions, some held in common with others, some unique to particular individuals. To understand the social world and the behaviour of individuals, he believed researchers would have to examine the formation and structure of the life experiences which give meaning to actions. As he said, "Meaning is a certain way of directing one's gaze at an item of one's own experience" (Schutz, 1972, 42).

The idea that experience could not be grasped as it occurs but only reflectively, once it has passed, is another of Schutz's important contributions to phenomenology. While it occurs, he postulated, behaviour is a "pre-phenomenal" experience. Behaviour has meaning because it is an experience that has occurred and has been looked at reflectively. The meaning does not, therefore, lie in the experience, because experiences can only be meaningful if they have been grasped reflectively. Consequently, not all experiences are meaningful because they are not all reflected upon. It is the act of the reflective glance that singles out elapsed experiences and endows them with meaning.

This theory has implications for interpretation, because it means that one cannot interpret another's experiences directly but only through picturing the other's reasons and motives. The interpretation of reasons and motives is based upon previous experience and on cultural inheritance, but the context is also extremely important. The interpreter may use her/his subjective meanings (and common-sense) to arrive at a reason for the other's action, or may try to find out what the other person means by putting her/himself into the place of the other and imagine selecting the same motives to thus understand why the particular actions were chosen. The social scientist should aim to comprehend the deeper levels of understanding, beyond ordinary conversation.

Schutz believed that the face-to-face orientation is the most important relationship, to which each participant brings a stock of knowledge. Like the other phenomenologists, Schutz agreed that this stock of knowledge, these "recipes" for action, are constantly revised during interaction with others and depending upon the context. This stock of knowledge contains ideal types which facilitate communication and which are indexical - that is they act as markers for whole sets of information and meanings. There is here a clear link with the concept of culture, outlined in chapter two. "Recipes for action" and an individual's stock of knowledge are culturally-determined. Thus, culture, through an individual's stock of knowledge, establishes recipes for action which enable individuals to know when they or others are ill, and the sort of behaviour that is expected of themselves or others who are defined as "ill".

Schutz was not only concerned with the theories of phenomenology, he also sought to outline an adequate methodology. He was aware that there is a danger that in observing the social behaviour of another person, the researcher may merely substitute her/his own ideal types for those in the mind of the subject. To avoid this, Schutz advocated a method which involved subjecting to detailed analysis everything that is normally taken for granted. Thus both the judgement of the researcher and the researched must be investigated so that the biases and prejudgements of both may be exposed and described. The role of the researcher is crucial here, with the requirement that she/he become immersed into the world of her/his subjects without preconceived ideas or theories, so that she/he can understand fully what the life of the other is like without relying on her/his own common-sense.

The task of the social sciences is seen by Schutz to be the understanding of the subjective meaning of social action. This is to to be achieved through the construction of ideal-types and second-order constructs. Second order constructs are similar to scientific constructs and are modelled on ideal typical situations. Critics of Schutz claim that the development of these second order constructs means that Schutz's theories are superficial (Hindess, 1972), and that they merely confirm the scientific method because they are concerned only with unquestioningly accepted behaviour (Gorman, 1975). Gorman claims that Schutz's ideal types and second order constructs fail when actors stop to think about situations because then actions are not merely products of social recipes. Gorman, however, unlike Schutz and his followers, fails to consider the importance of the context of the situation and to incorporate this in his analysis.

The importance of Schutz's work can be seen in the number of studies which rely to some extent upon his theories. Berger and Luckmann (1966), for example, draw heavily upon his work for their analysis of the social construction of reality, particularly his views on the origins and implications of common-sense knowledge. Others have also taken up the study of common-sense, showing how it can be rational and moral and so be an essential focus for social investigation (Silverman, 1972a). Others have developed Schutz's theory that each individual has a unique stock of knowledge, mostly handed down, but also dependent on previous experience, which leads the individual to experience the world through typifications, ideal types or recipes (Mennell, 1974; Silverman, 1972b).

Others still have attempted to develop methodologies from Schutz's suggestions. Walsh, (1972a, 34), for example, calls for a methodology from within the social world, one which depends upon the meanings used by members of society to categorise their activities - a theory, in other words, which "must start from the bottom and work up." Phillipson (1972b) has attempted to explain Husserl's method of "phenomenological reduction", the aim of which is to eliminate taken-for-granted beliefs and prejudgements and to uncover the intentional objects of consciousness. To do this, Phillipson argues, the researcher has to start with concrete experience, not theories, and concentrate on how members of society make sense of the social world. This can be accomplished through the use of long and detailed ethnographic descriptions and/or participant observation, combined with a detailed examination of the researcher's role and her/his own preconceptions and prejudices.

Methodological difficulties have, however, blunted the phenomenological critique. The critique proposes research which should focus on "the meaningful character of social phenomena" (Walsh, 1972a), but which also avoids "subjective excesses" (Louch, 1966). How to do research based on their theories has proved difficult for the phenomenologists. For some, the methodology should be left to the choice of the researcher, with the proviso that the technique should rest upon its ability to include the uniqueness of everyday life (Silverman, 1972c). Positivistic methods are rejected because they are seen to be based on unrecognised common-sense beliefs, tend to force the data into pre-conceived models and theories, and obscure the "sense" of the data by removing them from their contexts (Cicourel, 1964). The work of Schutz, adapted by others, calls upon the researcher to become fully conversant with her/his biographical situation and to tackle everything previously assumed within common-sense in order to get at the motives, thoughts, perceptions and meanings of the subjects being studied. This can be done through communication with the subject or subjects, usually by participant observation and/or detailed unstructured or semi-structured interviews (Douglas, 1971; Burgess, 1982), with the aim of studying the phenomena in their own terms and developing theories grounded in the data collected (Glaser and Strauss, 1967).

The work of Glaser and Strauss on grounded theory (1967) is worth considering here on its own merits. Their work is derived from phenomenology, but is concerned particularly with empirical work. "Grounded theory" is generated by empirical data which fits everyday situations and is understandable both to professional sociologists and lay people. Unlike positivistic research, grounded theory does not begin with theories and hypotheses to be tested, but consists of gathering qualitative data and at the same time the working out of hypotheses and concepts in relation to the data being collected. Work is started by a researcher choosing a topic, but, thereafter, the research is not guided, but is directed by what is discovered and logistical difficulties. Glaser and Strauss emphasise that there is no real clash between qualitative and quantitative methods, but that both are valid and should be treated equally, but according to different criteria.

Grounded theory is generated by comparative analysis, in which concepts which emerge from the data can be taken back to see if they are adequately representative. If the evidence changes, and a category no longer appears to "fit", the data can be examined to see why this might be the case, thus either explaining an unusual case or modifying the category to include the new information. This ties in with the notion of the negotiable nature of people's stocks of knowledge. Glaser and Strauss focus on the idea of verifying the theory, not through numbers or questions of adequacy, but by its relationship with the data and its comprehensibility.

Large amounts of data are required for grounded theory, and Glaser and Strauss suggest that methods such as participant observation, documentary analysis and ethnographic case studies will be the most suitable. The number of cases is not crucial because the "whole field" is not being tackled - the theory is attempting to describe and account for behaviour relevant to the theory. It is assumed that the research comes to a conclusion when sufficient data have been collected to saturate the categories or concepts and when the theory appears to fit most cases. The data should be presented in order that the reader may understand from where the categories have arisen. Grounded theory can be verified if it fits the empirical evidence from the area, is general enough to apply to many situations, and is relevant enough to make it applicable to the fluctuations of daily life (Glaser and Strauss, 1967).

The research in this thesis has its base in phenomenology. The phenomenological critique, particularly as developed by Schutz, emphasises the essential importance of studying phenomena in their own terms, without applying artificial constraints. Also emphasised is the need for the researcher to be able to empathise with the group under study while at the same time being critically aware of the influence she/he may be having on the research and on the group itself. In this study, the importance phenomenology places on the meanings of health and illness and of their negotiability depending upon each individual's personal and cultural heritage and in the context of everyday events is crucial. The concentration throughout is on the processes of experience, and the effects that common-sense and each individual's stock of knowledge may have on her/his choice of action are considered. Consequently, the research methods follow those of grounded theory (Glaser and Strauss, 1967) and the data are generated by in-depth interviews, organised into categories, and presented in depth to allow the reader's own assessment. Throughout the study, the emphasis is on the importance of being able to understand the world as the subjects see it, and to try to examine and take account of the researcher's own biases and common-sense view of the world.

Ethnomethodology

An offshoot from the phenomenological critique developed into a group of researchers known as the ethnomethodologists. Their focus of interest is on what goes on in everyday life, and they consider that common-sense and routines should be analysed closely. The basis of ethnomethodology comes from a fundamental idea that until we understand how we understand each other, all social enquiry is useless (Dreitzel, 1970). Ethnomethodologists such as Cicourel and Garfinkel tend to be interested in the language used by people in their everyday lives, and they have taken up and developed some of Schutz's ideas on the indexicality of expressions and accounts. Indexicality refers to the amount of shared background knowledge necessary to understand a particular phrase or message (Agar, 1980). Like the phenomenologists, their basic aim is to promote a better understanding of everyday life, particularly the ways in which sense or meaningfulness is established during the process of everyday interactions (Filmer, 1972).

According to Cicourel, actors in social situations attain a partial consensus on the meaning of some behaviour, but this consensus is not settled once and for all because it is negotiated (Dreitzel, 1970). The ethnomethodological focus here is the process by which actors manage to produce and sustain a sense of structure in everyday life. Since language is the principle medium of social interaction, it is language that should be looked at in detail. Some language is held in common and this is also considered in detail by ethnomethodologists (Walsh, 1972a). According to Phillipson (1972a), everyone is seen to have access to the social world through common-sense reasoning, and so in interaction we tend to assume that others know what we mean and will fill out what we say to make sense of it. This is the "inherent indexicality of accounts" - a sort of verbal shorthand. One of the aims of ethnomethodology, then, is better to understand the indexicality of language, not so that the indexical expressions can be changed, but so that the workings of society may be better understood.

Garfinkel advocates the use of various methods to get at these indexical expressions and common-sense meanings (Garfinkel, 1967). He suggests using tape-recorded interviews and participant observation so that discussions between participants may be analysed to reveal the nature of the language used; or using disruptive experiments in order to confuse routine activities and common-sense understandings so that they may be revealed and studied. As far as Garfinkel is concerned, everything taken for granted is problematic, and so he sees no superiority or inferiority in concepts. Consequently, unlike traditional sociologists, ethnomethodologists consider lay perceptions and opinions to be as valid as professional ideologies, and take as a subject for study the difference between public and private accounts of events (Cornwell, 1984).

Cicourel advocates the researcher deciding upon her/his own methodology to generate data. His only constraint is that the method must reveal the way in which members' theories combine with formal rules and practices, and expose the underlying patterns of social interaction. He was particularly concerned with, as he saw it, two types of rules held by everyone: basic rules, which are deep structures and enable the individual to make appropriate and even innovative responses to changing situations; and surface rules, which are shallow structures and constitute the tried and tested recipes used in everyday "normal" behaviour. Ethnomethodology should, therefore, study both types of rules - the surface ones which make up ordinary interaction, and the basic ones which give meanings and generate responses to the unexpected.

Ethnomethodology is of relevance to this study primarily because of its focus on everyday life and because its followers emphasis the comparable validity of lay and professional opinions and conceptions. In the field of health, this means that the neglected area of lay perceptions of health and illness can be considered as important as the dominant professional view of medicine. Some of Cicourel's ideas are also relevant, especially those concerning the use by individuals of surface and basic rules to cope with everyday life. In this study, it will be seen that the onset of unusual illnesses sometimes produces innovative responses arising from basic rules, whereas the incidence of "normal" illnesses such as colds and coughs can be coped with by using surface rules, and as part of everyday routines.

Symbolic Interactionism

Another sub-group of the interpretative school is based on the work of G.H. Mead and has developed the theory of symbolic interactionism. Again, the ultimate aim is to understand people's definitions and perceptions of reality, and, like the ethnomethodologists, symbolic interactionists concentrate particularly on the meanings and uses of language. The nature of "symbols" is crucial, and a symbol is taken to be a stimulus with a learned meaning (Rose, 1962). Behaviour arises from the response to a symbol, so the focus of concern for this group is on the shared characteristics of symbols (Walsh, 1972a).

The context within which an action takes place is also seen to be of importance, and so in any study of interaction, the researcher must analyse the action in its situation, and from the vantage point of the actor (Blumer, 1962). The symbolic interactionists emphasise the need to study society from the subject's point of view to discover the actor's definition and perception of reality (Schwartz and Jacobs, 1979). Hence Becker et al's study of a hospital and medical training from the students' point of view (Becker, 1961). "Culture" has been the subject of many studies with a symbolic interactionist perspective, mainly because culture is considered to be an elaborate set of meanings, values and symbols shared by a group, and which to some extent influences behaviour. It was believed that the learning of the culture of a group would enable people to predict other's behaviour (Rose, 1962).

Some of the basic principles of symbolic interactionism are shared with, and have been developed by, phenomenologists. In particular, the mechanistic and simplistic notion of behaviour as a pattern of stimulus and response has been criticised and dispensed with by the phenomenological critique. The techniques used by the symbolic interactionists are very similar to those of the phenomenologists: participant observation, documentary analysis, and ethnographic case studies; and it seems likely that the majority of researchers from this sub-school will become subsumed within the phenomenological/interpretative grouping.

ETHNOGRAPHY AND THE USE OF CASE STUDIES

Ethnography is part of a tradition labelled "naturalism" (Hammersley and Atkinson, 1983), which draws upon parts of symbolic interactionism, phenomenology, hermeneutics, linguistic philosophy and ethnomethodology. Ethnography is associated with the importance of understanding the perspectives of the people under study, and of observing their activities in everyday life (Hammersley and Atkinson, 1983). It emphasises that the researcher should be faithful to the phenomena under study rather than to particular methodological principles (Znanieki, quoted in Burgess, 1982). Ethnography has been used particularly in anthropological work, based upon the methods of participant observation, un- or semi-structured interviewing, or by the researcher becoming part of the society or social group being studied.

In traditional social science, the researcher holds all the power - she/he asks the questions, determines the categories of responses beforehand, decides on the time limits to the interview. In ethnography, however, it is the informant who has the power: ideally, the informant directs the interview, and the ethnographer becomes the learner, trying to understand what is happening and how situations connect with others (Agar, 1980). Often the ethnographer will represent her/himself as a student who wants to learn about a particular group or activity, emphasising that the informant is important and dominant (Agar, 1980).

The methodology of ethnography is usually dependent upon the constraints operating on whom or what the researcher wants to study. Initially, the ethnographer will try to gain access to the group chosen for study, either by approaching them through an intermediary, or without a prior introduction. The dress, appearance, accent, class, ethnicity, age and sex of both the informant and researcher are important here, and, unlike traditional social researchers, ethnographers do not, largely, ignore these issues. As Agar (1980) points out, the problem is not that biases exist, because they do exist in all types of social interaction, but how they can be documented and dealt with as part of the methodology. The effects of the researcher's personal characteristics, then, become an integral and beneficial part of the research (Easterday, 1982; Burgess, 1982).

After initial access is gained to the group under study, the next major problem is who is to be interviewed or observed? Ethnographers tend to use either non-probability methods of sampling, depending, for example, on who is available or to whom the researcher is introduced (Burgess, 1982); or theoretical sampling, in which the choice of informant is determined by theoretical development (Glaser and Strauss, 1967). Non-probability sampling may involve the researcher in actively choosing individuals who seem to be important, or may rely entirely upon chance or opportunity, or depend upon one informant passing the researcher onto others - snowball sampling (Honigmann, 1982). The use of "key informants" who are interviewed intensively over an extensive period and who may supply other informants is also a well-used sampling method in anthropological work (Tremblay, 1982).

Data are gathered in ethnographic research through interviews and/or observations that are recorded in the form of field notes and/ or audio or video tapes. Researchers may participate in the society they are studying in order to see how people interact. Participant observation means that the researcher must enmesh her/himself into the world being studied, yet at the same time, she/he must be aware of the effects she/he may be having on the people being studied (Schwartz and Jacobs, 1979). Un- or semi-structured interviews are often a major intrument used within participant observation, and they may also be used when adopting an "insider's perspective" is not possible.

The interview has been termed a "conversation with purpose" by Webb and Webb, 1932 (quoted by Burgess, 1982, 107). Un- or semi-structured interviews give the opportunity for researchers to probe deeply, and for informants to speak freely (Burgess, 1982). Ethnographers do not decide beforehand on the wording of the questions they want to ask, although they may well have a list of issues they want to cover, and they do not restrict themselves to a single mode of questioning (Hammersley and Atkinson, 1983). The interviewer becomes an active listener, building up rapport with the informant. Expressions of interest in statements, encouraging gestures, probing questions and leading questions are all part of the repertiore of un- and semi-structured interviewing (Agar, 1980). The researcher must again take note of the influence she/he may be having, but the method allows the validation of some stories by comparisons with others (Whyte, 1982).

It is also necessary for the ethnographer to be aware of the effects that taking notes or using a recording machine in front of informants may have. The data then have to be organised. It is considered essential, initially at least, to transcribe fully all tapes, even though this is a tedious and time-consuming business, because the aim of ethnography is to examine everything concerning the topic under consideration. Data can then be organised according to the researcher's interpretation of where there are "natural breaks", allowing the allocation of data to particular categories (Hammersley and Atkinson, 1983).

It must be emphasised that ethnographic research is a process which does not occur, like positivistic research, in linear stages, but is shaped by the data and their setting. The collection of data is not a distinct stage, but occurs throughout the development of theory, and is essential for the checking and validation of the theory. Typically, the research begins with a fairly wide view of the group or topic, and then the focus is progressively narrowed as the theory develops (Agar, 1980). Theory and method are, therefore, integrated and a fetishism with method is avoided (Burgess, 1982).

One of the major criticism of ethnographic work concerns the question of the representativeness of a small number of cases studied in detail. Case studies have, however, been part of social research for as long as it has existed, but the method was discredited in social science circles during the quantitative revolution after the second world war. The method has been particularly well used in anthropology, especially in the study of "exotic" cultures (see Wilson, 1951; Turner, 1957), where it has been used to attempt to interpret aspects of the way of life of groups of people.

Case studies were discredited principally because of the desire to quantify, and also because of the development of survey methods and sampling techniques based on statistical procedures. Since these techniques have been established, case studies have been subjected to assessment by the same criteria as for statistically-derived samples, even though this betrays a confusion between the procedures (Mitchell, 1983). Questions about the validity of making inferences from a small number of cases have been asked, for example. Mitchell (1983) answers this challenge by showing that the inferences from statistics are based on correlations and are linked together by theoretical thinking; whereas inferences from case studies are logical or causal and are based in the data collected.

Statistical inferences, based on correlations, do not explain associations between variables, only declare that a relationship may occur according to a particular probability. It may be that in some cases the presence of a strong correlation does not necessarily ensure that a causal relationship does exist between variables. Inferences from statistical samples require two steps: firstly statistical inference, which makes a statement about the confidence one may have in a relationship, and secondly, the logical inference, which draws conclusions about the links between the data and a set of theoretical principles (Mitchell, 1983). In case studies, only the second step is necessary.

The major characteristic of case studies is that they capture the "wholeness" of an individual or group. They can be focused on an individual through the life history approach or on a group, but they are located in a wider context which should be taken into account. The case-study approach has been adapted from medical science, where the detailed analysis of an individual case is used to develop more general theoretical statements (Becker in Sills, 1968; Eckstein, 1975). A case becomes of particular importance when it is set against a knowledge of the background, and the extent to which generalisations may be made from case studies depends upon the adequacy of the underlying theory, rather than on the case itself (Mitchell, 1983).

The interpretation of cases involves some simplification of the complexity and detail present in the data. A major advantage of the method is the depth of knowledge it gives to the researcher of particular social processes. Each case is compared with the emergent theory, and any cases that contradict the theory are examined closely. The researcher then aims to discover why such cases are unique, and whether or not the theory needs to be changed. Hence cases, clearly argued, may illuminate the workings of the social system (Gluckman, 1961), so long as they are only used analytically if embedded in an appropriate theoretical framework (Mitchell, 1983), and are considered situationally, in context (Van-Velsen, 1967).

Ethnographic methods and case studies are integral parts of the research in this thesis. For the empirical work, a combination of non-probability sampling methods has been employed. Key informants were used initially, one from each of the Afro-Caribbean and Asian groups, in order to find out some details about the groups and to discover the best ways to approach other informants. The key informants were seen regularly during the year of empirical work. After they were located, the snowball sampling technique was used: they provided introductions to their friends and/or relatives, some of whom, in turn, led to others willing to be involved. The method meant that the informants were seen when they were willing, that they always had prior notice, and that they usually knew at least one other informant who had already been interviewed.

The data were gathered using semi-structured interviews. All informants were asked to give details of health and illness during their lives, and the order of points to be discussed was flexible, depending on the direction of informants. The list of questions usually asked of the informants during the life-story interviews is contained in Appendix I. Some individuals were also asked about more focused issues on a separate occasion, and these were determined by answers to the first set of interviews. These issues are reproduced in Appendix II. All of the interviews were tape-recorded and fully transcribed. The focus throughout on individuals as case-studies is the result of the aim to capture the wholeness and uniqueness of individuals. The research was carried out according to the ethnographic pattern of collecting data, formulating theory and cross-checking information contemporaneously.

Conclusion

The methodology of the empirical research in this thesis is, therefore, derived from phenomenology and ethnography. There is, however, one glaring omission from these theories: a consideration of the power base of society. This is of crucial importance for the present project, and so radical theories are drawn upon to outline the background and context within which black people live in Britain (see chapter one). The study is set within this context, and is based on case studies which focus upon the perceptions and experiences of health and illness of individuals.

The topic of black people's health is one which in particular has needed a new approach. Several policy initiatives in Britain, based upon positivistic research done by medical experts without consulting black people, have failed and have caused and are still causing great offence (see the rickets controversy, chapter three). It has been shown that there are great disjunctions between lay and professional views about health and illness (Freidson, 1970a; Dingwall, 1976; Cornwell, 1984), and these are brought particularly into focus when the lay group has a different cultural heritage from both the professionals and the lay group usually taken to be the norm. It is known that the majority of ill-health is dealt with outside the professional sphere (Eisenberg and Kleinman, 1981; see also Chapter two), particularly within the family (Robinson, 1971), and so it would seem to be essential that research should be grounded here, at the individual level and within the family.

Service providers need to know what to expect of their patients and what the patients expect of them, but calls for research to determine what black people as a whole think will fail because black people are not a homogeneous group. Each individual has unique ways of perceiving the world and acting upon the information she/he receives. Consequently, the need is to understand exactly what is going on in the lives of a small number of people, and once this is known, some general principles may emerge which may be applicable outside the small group. A study has been undertaken in Australia concerning the perceptions and experiences of health and illness of a group of Aborigines which has shown this to be possible and worthwhile (Nathan and Leichleitner-Japanangka, 1983). There is a need for a greater understanding of lay perceptions and experiences of health and illness of black people in Britain, and how these perceptions and experiences fit into the social context. This is the aim of the empirical work outlined in the next two chapters.

PART II
THE EMPIRICAL WORK

Introduction

INTRODUCTION

This section outlines the way in which the empirical work was undertaken. As indicated in chapter four, the field research draws upon the methodology of interpretative sociology, particularly phenomenology and ethnography. The research did not begin with the formulation of hypotheses to be tested as in the positivist tradition; after the initial definition of the topic of interest, the processes of collecting and analysing the data were undertaken at the same time. It was decided at an early stage that the focus of interest would be on perceptions and experiences of health, and that it was important to consider this topic among the neglected black population. Since people of Asian and Afro-Caribbean descent make up a large proportion of the black population living in Britain, they were the groups chosen for study.

A review of the literature concerning the health and illness of the black population has revealed several biases and omissions (see chapter three). The race relations literature (see chapter one), showed that black people are discriminated against in almost all sections of society, and yet there have been few attempts to link this work with their health. The studies of black people's health that have been undertaken tend to focus almost exclusively on illnesses or diseases that are unusual or that can be attributed to people's habits or diets (see chapter three). In many cases, the different cultural heritages of black people have been invoked and their cultures, personal or religious habits have been blamed for ill-health or levels of disadvantage (see chapters two and three). Finally, few researchers have listened to what the people involved have to say and tried to understand their point of view. These are perhaps the most obvious gaps in the literature, and the ones that this thesis seeks to begin to fill.

As indicated in the preface and chapter four, ethnographic and interpretative sociological work take the role of the researcher to be crucial. It is known that the researcher has prejudices and preconceptions, and it is important for these to be known to the reader so that she/he may see why certain interpretations are made. For this purpose, a short autobiography is offered.

I was born in Cheltenham, UK, in 1960. Both my parents were born in London. My father's family are of distant Irish origin, and my mother is Jewish. According to tradition, Jewish ethnicity is passed from mother to children, and so I am ethnically Jewish. I have never practised Judaism, but my ethnicity is very important to me. My experiences of anti-semitism throughout my life have convinced me of the largely racist nature of British society and made me a passionate anti-racist.

My father died in 1961, and so I was brought up in a one-parent family. I can see advantages and disadvantages in this form of family structure. I went to a state (grammar) school, and thence to Liverpool University for a BA (Hons) degree in geography. After Liverpool, I moved to east London to undertake a Ph.D at Queen Mary College. Despite my education, I do not consider myself to be part of the "middle-class", nor can I claim to be "working class". I feel, then, "classless", and somewhat of an outsider. I am politically left-wing and a lacto-vegetarian (I do not eat meat, but still eat dairy products and, rarely, fish).

These matters should be borne in mind during the reading of the empirical work. Of particular importance to this project was the empathy between the informants and myself, in part because of my ethnicity, in part because I was prepared to listen to them. Other biographical details became significant when the informants and I discussed matters such as family members and structures, numbers of children, bereavement, class, racism, education and food.

An attempt was made to use a questionnaire for the study based largely on the General Household Survey, but the questions contained in this were found to be too rigid and inflexible to elicit details on perceptions of health and illness. Some of the structured questions may also be ethnocentric (Cicourel, 1964), because they have not been designed with members of particular ethnic groups in mind. It was also found that the strict and inflexible order of the questions tended to inhibit the discussion of particular episodes or events, and to break up the telling of stories, thus losing much relevant material.

Ethnography and the case study method (see chapter four) typically utilise participant observation or semi- or un-structured interviews as the means of generating data. In this study of black people's health by a white, albeit Jewish, woman, it was felt that semi- or un-structured interviews would be most suitable. The time necessary for a white researcher to "infiltrate" a black social network was not available to the project, since it was necessary to complete the field work within one year. Participant observation also demands, if it is done well, that the researcher should live with the subjects, and learn as much about their lives as possible. In this project, the aim was to focus upon health and illness, and so such detail was not considered necessary.

Semi-structured discussions with the subjects, where the researcher has a list of points to be covered, but allows the informant to speak freely, were considered much more suitable. Each informant was "interviewed" at least once, and several more than once. The first meeting and discussion with an informant was aimed at allowing the informants to talk about their perceptions and experiences of health, illness and the health services throughout their lives, beginning with their childhoods and ending with the present. The order of the questions was determined by the responses of the informants and the degree of rapport between the interviewer and the interviewee. After these "life-story" interviews were undertaken with several informants, a list of points to be covered was drawn up. These questions were normally, but not always asked of each informant, and are reproduced in Appendix I. The basic content of Appendix I is designed for the Afro-Caribbean women. The points marked with an asterisk contain information on menstruation, pregnancy and ante-natal which were not used with men. Some additional questions were asked of the women of Asian descent - these are bracketed in Appendix I and concern issues of language.

The interviews began with my asking the informants about their health during their childhoods, and from then on, my aim was to prompt the informants into talking, in detail, about health and illness throughout their lives. I intervened to ask questions only if it seemed that the informants had finished a story or were moving too far from the central issues of health and illness.

As soon as each interview was completed, the tapes were fully transcribed. Once the first five had been transcribed and read through, it was clear that the data had to be broken up to allow comparisons and analysis. Several topics of common-ground were clearly evident: especially those concerning work, hospitals, remedies and GPs, for example. These comparable discrete sections of interviews are known as categories (see chapter four) and they can be removed from the totality of the interviews to allow comparisons with other informants. In the life-story discussions, these categories are partly chronological: childhood, adolescence and migration, the future; partly concerned with health: pregnancy, present health, recent health, remedies, other people's health, NHS doctors and drugs, private medicine, hospitals; partly political: racism, the government, housing, work; and there are some miscellaneous categories: food, smoking, exercise and religion.

Each of the transcripts was carefully analysed, and sections, stories or statements by informants referring to particular categories were copied and placed into category files. Some stories and statements were relevant to more than one category, and they were entered fully in each category-file each time. The context of the answer was always noted, since context is essential for the understanding of statements. When sixteen informants of Afro-Caribbean and fourteen informants of Asian descent had been interviewed, the material was written up in prose form (see, for example, Donovan, 1983).

It was clear from these reports that some points of interest had been only touched upon, and that other matters had been suggested, but not confirmed during the life-story interviews. It was felt necessary, therefore, to return to some of the informants, this time for more focused talk. The framework of this talk is reproduced in Appendix II. Again, the order and form of the "questions" were not set, but could vary according to the informant's responses. Most of the questions were asked of each individual, although the points concerning hot and cold are particularly designed for Asian informants. There was no appreciable difference between the questions asked of the women and men.

The analysis of these interviews was similar to that outlined for the life-story data. The interviews were all fully transcribed and then read through to identify any discrete topics in the material. Categories were this time organised in terms of: fate, fault, definitions of health, illness and perfect health, heredity, germs and viruses, incurable conditions, psychological effects of ill-health, living in Britain, racism, religion, hot and cold, food, and weight. Once organised into categories, the material was again written up in continuous prose form.

The study is concerned with thirty informants: ten women and six men of Afro-Caribbean descent, and fourteen women of Asian descent. All thirty were interviewed at length at least once, the life-story interview lasting between forty minutes and two-and-three-quarter hours. One informant from each of the two ethnic groups became key informants who were seen on many occasions and who introduced me to other informants. Ten people (three women and three men of Afro-Caribbean descent and four women of Asian descent) were also asked the more focused questions, taking between thirty minutes and one-and-a-half hours. No-one was visited without their prior knowledge of my arrival and purpose.

All the material was re-read before the final writing up commenced. In this thesis, all the speech between quotation marks is copied faithfully from tape-recorded comments, and is represented as it was spoken, phonetically where necessary. The words and phrases, "you know", "like", "sort of", and "um" have been largely left out because they tend to disrupt the flow of the narrative. Three full stops (...) are used to denote that non-essential sections larger than a phrase such as "you know" have been omitted. Bracketed phrases [] have been added where appropriate to explain indefinite articles used by informants, to guide the reader, to explain dialect words, or to help the flow of the narrative.

For the convenience of the reader, the empirical work has been broken into three sections. Chapter five concerns the data from the informants of Afro-Caribbean descent. Chapter six contains the data from the informants of Asian descent. Chapter seven consists of an examination of the similarities and differences between the two groups, and contains a critical assessment of the value of the research.

5 The perceptions and experiences of the Afro-Caribbean informants

The Informants

As explained in chapter four, informants were obtained according to the key informant and snowball sampling stategies. The first five informants were contacted via the workplace of a fellow (part-time) research student in October, 1982. The research student introduced me to Ivy, Delores, Millie, Ruby and Judy, and they all agreed to be interviewed at a later date. Ivy was interviewed at work, in a private room, but all the others were seen in their own homes. Delores was the most forthcoming and helpful of the five, and she became the key informant of the Afro-Caribbean group.

Delores was visited on many occasions during the year of empirical work, and she gave a great deal of advice as to who should be interviewed and which questions might be inappropriate, and she suggested some questions that I had failed to include early on. Delores treated me as a student who needed her help, and she was very willing to give it, and extremely keen to talk about the issues of health and illness. "It's about time the people up there took a listen to us", she said at an early meeting. The relationship between Delores and myself was very much like the adult-child relationship often found in ethnographic research (Agar, 1980).

Ivy, Delores and Ruby were all seen in October, 1982. Millie was interviewed in November, and Judy some time later in February, 1983, because of her position as a temporary worker who was not always available. The five women all work in the same old people's home, as care assistants, except for Millie who is a laundry worker. Their position as care-assistants means that they look after old and often sick people on a day-to-day basis, and so they have an acute awareness of some health issues. This has to be taken into account when their answers are analysed.

After her "life-story" interview, Delores insisted that I should interview two of her sons, Leroy and Carlton, who were both willing to talk to me. The snowball sampling began here. Leroy and Carlton then introduced me to their friend, Earl. Earl suggested that I should interview his parents, Joe and Jean, and his brothers, Danny and Paul, who were also introduced to me (see Fig 5(i)).

The life-story interviews with Leroy and Carlton occurred in December, 1982. Joe, Jean, Danny and Paul were all seen in January, 1983. After these were completed, I started to interview the women of Asian descent (see chapter six). In September, 1983, however, I made contact with a separate group of people of Afro-Caribbean descent. Martha was interviewed first, introduced to me by a friend of a friend, and then her next-door neighbour, Emily, was interviewed. Louise was also interviewed in September, 1983: she is a friend of Emily's. The last interview in this group was in October, 1983, with Donna, Delores's daughter, who was originally supposed to have been seen the year before, but who had been unavailable because of personal difficulties.

The relationships of the informants are set out in Fig 5(i). Some biographical details are contained in Tables 5(i) and 5(ii). Thirteen of the people of Afro-Caribbean descent were born outside Britain: Ivy, Ruby, Joe, Jean and Judy in Jamaica; Delores, Leroy, Carlton, Martha and Donna in Barbados; Millie and Emily in Ghana; and Louise in Dominica. Earl, Danny and Paul were born in Britain. The women are aged between 24 and 58 years; the men between 21 and 57 years.

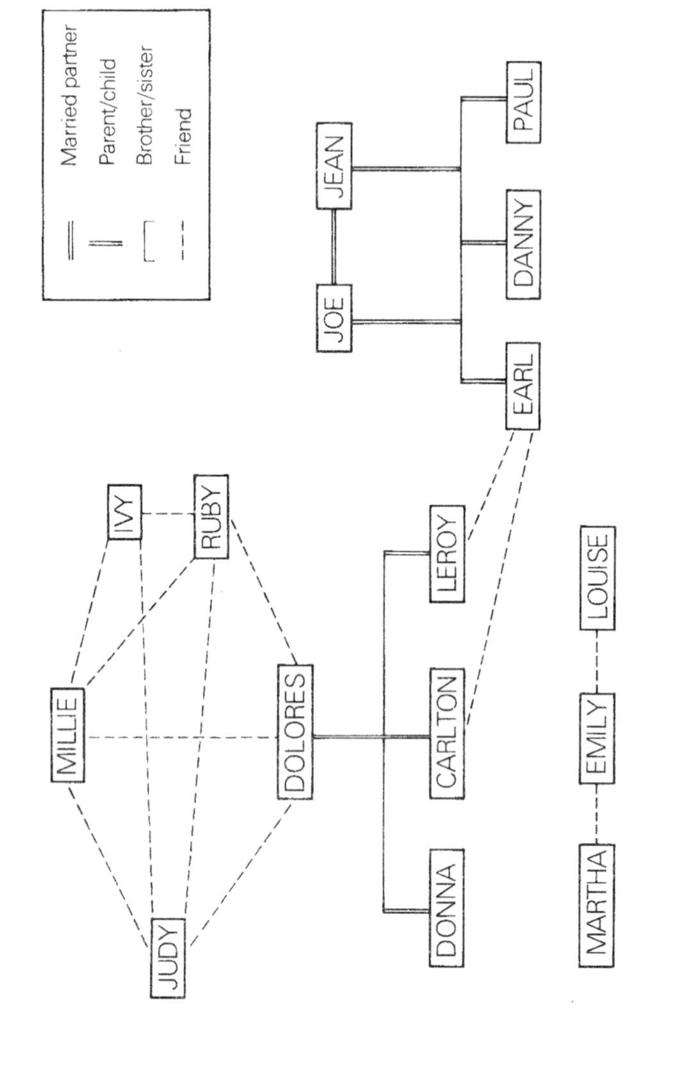

Fig5(i) **Relationships of Informants**

Table 5(i) Some Biographical Details of the Informants

NAME	PLACE OF BIRTH	AGE	MARITAL STATUS*	NUMBER OF CHILDREN
Ivy	Jamaica	43	M	5
Ruby	Jamaica	51	D	2
Delores	Barbados	51	D,RM	5
Leroy	Barbados	22	S,CH	1
Carlton	Barbados	21	S	0
Donna	Barbados	26	S	1
Joe	Jamaica	57	M	5
Jean	Jamaica	58	M	6
Earl	U.K.	23	S,CH	2
Paul	U.K.	24	S	0
Danny	U.K.	25	S	0
Judy	Jamaica	24	S	2
Millie	Ghana	34	S	3 (+2)**
Martha	Barbados	49	M	6
Emily	Ghana	36	S	0
Louise	Dominica	49	Sep	0

Notes

* Marital status S = single Sep = separated
M = married D = divorced
RM = remarried CH = co-habiting
W = widowed

** Millie has three children of her own and looks after two of her sister's.

Table 5(ii) Some More Biographical Details of the Informants

NAME	JOB	PARTNER'S JOB *	HOUSE TYPE**	LENGTH OF INTERVIEW	SECOND INTERVIEW
Ivy	Care Assistant	BR Fitter	MH	1hr20m	no
Ruby	Care Assistant		CF	2hr45m	no
Delores	Care Assistant	BR Fitter	CF	2hr30m	yes
Leroy	Scaffolder		CF	1hr20m	yes
Carlton	Factory work		CF	1hr15m	yes
Donna	Clerk		MF	- 45m	no
Joe	BR Fitter	Tea lady	MH	1hr -	no
Jean	Tea lady	BR Fitter	MH	- 40m	no
Earl	Maintenance Engineer		CF	1hr10m	yes
Paul	Insurance Seller		MH	- 45m	no
Danny	Toolmaker		MH	1hr -	no
Judy	Care Assistant (Temp)		CF	1hr -	no
Millie	Laundry and Cleaner		CF	1hr30m	no
Martha	Cleaner	Bus Driver	CF	1hr -	yes
Emily	------		CF	1hr -	yes
Louise	------		CF	1hr -	no

Notes

* Husband/wife or co-habitee, where applicable.

** H = house F = flat/maisonette

M = mortgaged C = council rented

There are some important details not contained in Tables 5(i) and (ii). Ivy, for example, was the only informant not to be interviewed in her own home. She was initially fairly skeptical about the interview and aware of the tape-recorder, but once she got going, she enjoyed telling her life-story.

Delores and Ruby are close friends, and share many views on health and illness. Both spent very little time discussing their childhoods, being much more concerned with the present or recent past. On many occasions both women told very long and detailed stories, sometimes only loosely connected with the original question, and for long periods I said very little, if anything.

The interviews with Millie and Judy were not so free-flowing. Both women are young single parents who work, and so have very little time to spare. One of Millie's children also has sickle-cell anaemia, and so from time to time requires special attention. Interviews with both women tended to focus on a single or a couple of issues. For Millie, this was the poor treatment she received at several local hospitals; for Judy, it was the worries about the futures of her children and her difficult housing conditions. Donna's interview was similarly concerned with her worries about her daughter's future and her mother's (Delores's) ill-health.

The interviews with the men (Leroy, Earl, Carlton, Danny, Paul and Joe) were much easier than expected. They did not seem to mind talking about their perceptions and experiences of health and illness, and Joe, Leroy and Carlton had a great deal to say, despite their very limited experience of ill-health. Joe has some very well-worked out theories of how the body works, based on his own experiences. The interview with Earl was disturbed by his younger son (fourteen months) crawling over us and the tape-recorder!

Jean and Martha were quite difficult to talk to. Both declared that they had few, if any, illnesses, and so had very little to say. Jean gave single-sentence answers to many of the points put to her, and was reluctant to theorise about health and ill-health. Martha had a similar attitude to questions about her own few experiences of ill-health, but some questions produced lengthy stories and reams of material.

Martha introduced me to her next-door neighbour, Emily. Emily was easy to interview and difficult to leave. She is very lonely because she has been unable to leave her flat very often after recent episodes of severe ill-health. Her friend, Louise, has also experienced several episodes of severe ill-health, and is similarly house-bound. Louise's interview was made difficult for me by her strong French West Indian accent, but simple questions often led her to tell long and involved stories about her life and health.

During the interviews I tried to be aware of the effects I might be having on the responses of the informants. Throughout the interviews, I emphasised that I was a student who wanted to know what ordinary black people felt and thought about their health, and to understand how they coped with episodes of ill-health. At no stage did I hide my intention only to interview black people, and when asked why, I always explained about the poverty of good research in the field, and the failure of others to listen to the views of ordinary people. On several occasions I was asked about my own background, and again I always told as much as I could. They were particularly interested in my Jewish background and my father's early death.

I asked some of those interviewed whether they thought it would have been better if I had been black, and they all said that they did not think it made any difference. Delores even suggested that it was better that I was white because I would, therefore, be better able to make their views heard by those who could alter policies. I think, however, that my not being black did affect some answers, particularly those on race questions, although my being Jewish did seem to alleviate some of these difficulties. When we exchanged stories about racism, for example, some of them said that they thought the experience must be worse for Jews because their identitiy is not always obvious, and so they hear what people really think, whereas it is obvious if you are black and so people avoid you rather than declare their feelings. Several felt the failure of whites to look them in the eyes was particularly offensive.

Some of the informants mentioned that they had "been done" by surveys before, but felt that they had not been given the freedom to offer their own opinions. On many, many occasions, long and detailed stories, conveying just the material I wanted, came from fairly basic questions, such as, "How would you describe your health at the moment?" or "Do you like working?" which just set people off. The interview then progressed something like normal conversation, and both of us could relax. Many of the informants said that they had enjoyed the experience.

The use of the tape-recorder did affect some of the informants, at least initially. Once they were telling stories, however, it seemed that the majority forgot that it was there. Once an informant was in full flow, even the replacement of a tape sometimes went unnoticed. Emily and Carlton were the only ones to ask if they could hear their own tapes. Everybody asked what would happen to the tapes, but on being told that they were only an aid to me instead of note-taking, that I would be the only person to listen to them, and that in anything I wrote their names would be changed, nobody objected to the use of tapes or the tape-recorder.

The focused questions were asked of six members of this group. Delores, as the key informant, was the first to answer them, and she and my fellow part-time research student endeavoured to involve the others who had been in the first round. Unfortunately, several were unable to be interviewed again. Ruby had retired, and was spending several months in Jamaica. Ivy and Louise were too ill. Judy had moved, and left her job at the old people's home. Joe, Jean, Danny and Paul could not be contacted. Consequently, the focused questions were asked of Delores, Leroy, Carlton, Earl, Martha and Emily. These interviews took place between October, 1983 and January, 1984, and lasted between thirty minutes, and one hour and thirty minutes.

By the time of the final contact, some of the informants' circumstances had changed. Leroy had moved out of his parents' home into a nearby flat with his girlfriend and their son. Carlton lost his job at the record manufacturer's and had been unemployed for about a month. Emily had almost recovered from her operation, was getting out much more, and had enrolled at the local college.

The material from the focused questions adds to and builds upon the data from the life-history interviews, and so they have been combined and the analysis written up as a whole. The material has been broken into categories as suggested by the data itself (see chapter four). There are seven broad sections into which the categories fall and are reported. These concern an outline of the informants' health life-histories; the perceptions and definitions of health and ill-health; the causes of ill-health and the role of individual responsibility in this; the perceived severity of conditions and exacerbatory factors; a general section including the effects of what might loosely be called "culture" on lifestyle and ultimately health; the effects that living in Britain have on health; and their experiences of the health services. These are reported, below. An outline of the ill-health histories of selected informants is shown in Table 5(iii).

Table 5(iii) Outline of the major illness/disease events of selected informants' lives

NAME	SURGERY	SERIOUS ILL-HEALTH	MINOR ILL-HEALTH
Ivy		Hypertension	Dislocated knee (work injury)
Ruby	Hysterectomy	Sugar diabetes Asthma High blood pressure	Dislocated shoulder (work injury)
Delores	Hysterectomy	High blood pressure	Eye infection and back injury (both work injuries)
Leroy			Groin strain (work injury)
Joe		Ulcer Nervous breakdown	
Earl			Upset stomach (work illness)
Danny			Cuts (work injuries)
Judy			Eye infection (work injury)
Millie	Hysterectomy		Headaches
Martha		Thyroid trouble	
Emily	Hysterectomy	Anaemia	'Flu
Louise	Mastectomy Hysterectomy		

Health and Illness in Their Lifetimes : An Introduction

All the informants were asked about their health and the ill-health they had suffered during their childhood and teenage years, but none of them wanted to discuss these in any detail. Of much greater importance to everyone were the health worries of the present or illnesses of the more recent past. The teenage years seemed largely non-existent: most of the women, especially, went from childhood to adulthood without a stage of transition, usually by becoming mothers. The childhood years appear to be too distant, with informants saying, for example, "I can't remember" (Ivy), or, "I don't know" (Millie). Very few illnesses are reported during these years.

Most of the informants say that they had very healthy childhoods. Ruby had asthma which seemed to her to run in the family. Some could remember having childhood illnesses such as chickenpox or measles. Carlton and Earl remember that they often had asthma, bronchitis and colds when they were young, caused, they believe, by factories and housing conditions. In the West Indies, doctors charge for visits, and as all the informants who were brought up there came from relatively poor backgrounds, doctors were rarely seen. Consequently, there was a vast array of home remedies, usually dispensed by the oldest woman in the household, and some of which have been retained for use in Britain. Even those born in Britain speak of their mothers using home remedies to cure their "everyday" illnesses. Only the two from Ghana do not mention remedies specifically, although Millie does speak of her mother using "bush" cures. Delores says, for example: "We didn't used to go to no doctors 'cause our parents used to go to the field and pick de bush. Our mother would dry them and boil dat bush and we'd drink it, and that would get into our blood and that heals up."

Hospitals were rarely used by the informants, except in emergencies after accidents such as Joe falling off a horse, Carlton being knocked down on a pedestrian crossing and Paul falling on a dustbin. The men remember their teenage years as times of great enjoyment and very good health, apart from sports injuries and colds or 'flu. The teen years are also remembered by the women as being healthy, and most of them had their first children during these years. Only Louise and Emily have not had children.

Pregnancy and childbirth are not treated as anything but part of the natural order of things by the women, and none of them has any regrets about becoming mothers. Ivy had two children in Jamaica and three in Britain; Delores had all five in Barbados (she had another that died); Ruby had both of hers in Britain; Millie had two in Ghana and one in Britain; Jean had one in Jamaica and five in Britain; Judy had two in Britain; Martha had four in Barbados and two in Britain; and Donna had her one in Britain. All had some sort of medical help during their pregnancies: a doctor or a clinic for the pregnancy and a hospital delivery for those in Britain; and usually a doctor to check on the pregnancy, but then a midwife and occasionally a doctor "in case" for the deliveries which were usually at home in the Caribbean or Ghana. None of the women who were pregnant in Britain attended ante-natal classes: the younger women were not aware of them, and the older women felt they were experienced enough not to need them.

A time that is not remembered with pleasure is the period of migration and settlement in Britain. Only Danny, Paul and Earl were born here - all the others arrived during the late 1950s to 1970s. Donna, Carlton and Leroy came aged between five and nine years to join their parents, after first their father and then Delores had moved to Britain to settle beforehand. Martha, Louise, Ruby and Jean all arrived in Britain after their husbands had found jobs and houses. Millie and Ivy came to get jobs. Judy came to join her parents, and Emily to live with an uncle. Joe came to get a job after the friend to whom he had lent money had made arrangements for him.

Carlton, Leroy, Donna and Judy can remember very little about the journey and arrival. Of the others, only Martha and Joe thought the experience a pleasant one: "I didn't find it hard. I came to join my husband ... Everything was provided for me" (Martha); "It was all set up ... It was cold, but it was all right" (Joe). The shock of the cold weather is mentioned by several: "When I come here, I didn't understand what cold was, because if I did, I wouldn't have come" (Louise); "I got here on Christmas night. It was pouring with snow ... If I coulda got on the plane, I'd go back that night!" (Delores). For Ivy and Millie, their expectations of Britain were quickly shattered: "When we came to Britain, we were British. In those days, Britain was called the mother country, so you were expecting a motherly reception, but it wasn't like that at all" (Ivy); "When I reach the airport, I regret it. When I was comin', the way you hear about Britain, you think it's heaven or somethin', but when you come, is different altogether" (Millie). The initial shock of arrival was tempered by some by the availability of jobs, and as Ivy says, "As the years go by, you get used to it ... You sorta accept what's goin' on."

This, then, is the background to their arrival in Britain. The majority of interviews were, however, taken up with the concerns of the present and the recent past, and so these are considered in detail below. Although the material has been broken into sections, it is important to bear in mind that many of the issues raised are interlinked and often intricately related.

Perceptions of Health and Illness

Definitions of health

Health is seen to be a residual state by most of the informants. It is seen as the normal functioning of the body, the pristine state before illness sets in. Health is not really a state that is easy to define, and its absence is much more obvious than its presence. All the informants agree that good health is important to them, and essential for them to carry out their lives: "If you've not got your health, you don't enjoy life" (Danny); "If your health isn't good, well, you're no good for anything - you can't help yourself. Like, I'm workin', and I need my health" (Martha); "If I'm not healthy, I've got no-one to look after the kids" (Millie); and, "Health is very important. I like workin'. If you're sick, you can't work" (Joe). Throughout the interviews, the importance of health is linked with present-day concerns such as work, child-care and happiness, and often the specific relevance of an illness will be weighed against these issues.

Most of the informants believe that there is such a thing as "perfect health" - in theory, at least, if not in practice. Carlton, for example, believes that perfect health is the state of the very young which is eroded by time and the conditions in Britain. He says, "I had it [perfect health] when I was younger. I haven't got it now. It happen to you in this country. I don't think you can get perfect health over here." Delores and Martha also believe in the perfect health of the young, Delores saying that, "You start OK, but then you go down." Delores continues, and says of herself: "I haven't been, like, very ill in my life, but I haven't had perfect health. Everyone gets something."

Earl and Emily believe that the concept of "perfect health" includes "minor, niggly things like coughs and colds which everybody gets" (Earl), or, "a few allergies" (Emily). If these are disregarded, "Then you could say you were in perfect health" (Earl). Leroy is less convinced than some of the others about the existence of perfect health, particularly, "in this day and age" with all the, "chemicals and stuff about." Perfect health is not something that any of the informants believe they have, but this does not necessarily preclude its existence, particularly when they have memories of childhood where, they believe, no-one was ill.

The health of the informants at the time of the life-story interview varies from, "Fine" (Donna), to, "Not good enough. I think it's fading" (Delores). For most of them, their health is, "OK" (Carlton), or, "All right" (Leroy). On the whole, these are the people who have no current episodes of ill-health. For those who are currently, or have been recently, ill, the picture is somewhat different: Emily, for example, says: "Recently, I have been very ill" (Emily). "Health" is again seen principally in terms of the presence or absence of illness or disease.

Definitions of Ill-Health

Several words in English are used to denote the presence of ill-health: illness and disease are the most commonly used, and sickness is an alternative term. During the life-story interview, the informants gave some indication of what they meant by these terms, and in the focused talk, they were asked specifically what the terms meant to them, and what distinguished one from another.

Ill-health is normally defined by what it stops a person doing, and this is particularly important for those with jobs and/or child-care duties: ill- health is, "Somethin' that stop me from doin' what I am able to do, which puts me down, makes me feel sick, feel weak" (Carlton); "Anything that keeps me off work for a period of two or three days" (Earl); "You can't carry on to do your work, to clean the house" (Delores). For others, it is a perception that, "You feel that there is something wrong with you in your body, you just don't feel up to the day" (Emily). Martha finds it hardest of all to define ill-health, because, she says, "Like, I've never experienced anybody, like, really ill in my family", and because of this, she feels she cannot really speak about it.

"Illness" and "disease" are concepts which refer to particular types of ill-health. "Illness" is the more general description, being applied to conditions such as, "a cold or an upset stomach" (Earl). Delores and members of her family share a conception of "illness" and "<u>real</u> illness". Illness here includes colds, aches and pains - all things which are minor, and which if, "You can work and carry on, well you carry it [the minor illnesses]" (Delores). <u>Real</u> illness, on the other hand, is, "When you are a bed patient. That's an illness, say a <u>heavy</u> illness" - one that actually stops an individual from doing what she/he normally does.

"Disease" is another specific concept which relates to particular forms of ill-health, and it is seen to be quite distinct from "illness": "An illness is gonna go away, but a disease is gonna be there for a real good time. A disease I would take to myself much stronger than an illness. I might think, 'I've got a disease, that means it's gonna last a certain amount of time, or it might last for a good time.' An illness, well, I can recover from an illness - no problem!" (Carlton); "Well, you can be, like, seriously ill and get over it, but ... a disease like you can really die of. It's two different things" (Leroy); "When you've got a disease, you've gotta carry it. You can never get rid of it ... It quiets down, yeah, but you can be sure it'll come back again, 'cause it's there" (Delores); "An illness can go, but a disease is something that you can't cure" (Emily).

Disease is also seen as something which has a particular cause. Martha believes that diseases are largely hereditary, and her family experience bears this idea out: five generations are still alive, and no-one has ever had what she considers to be <u>real</u> illness: a disease. Emily thinks illnesses are temporary things like 'flu or headache, whereas diseases are recurrent complaints like asthma and bronchitis. Earl also sees illnesses as temporary phenomena which interfere with the daily routine, like his stomach upset, whereas a disease is something like his girlfriend's psoriasis.

The informants said, generally, that they were last ill quite a long time before the life-story interview. None of them fitted into the GHS and other social survey's definitions of "acute" ill-health, because none was ill in the two weeks before the interview. Typically, they were last ill a few months before the interview, or said that they could not remember when they were last ill. The most commonly mentioned illness was 'flu (Emily, Carlton and Paul). Others mentioned include accidents at sport or work (Ivy, Delores, Leroy), a stomach upset (Earl), or headaches (Millie). The others could not specify a time when they were last unwell. Louise says, for example: "At times, I feel, like today, may be I feel not well ... Tomorrow I feel better."

The first indication that a person is not well is usually, "a feelin'. Something out of the ordinary" (Delores). For Emily, it is, "When you are not in your usual self. That means the body is tellin' you there is somethin' wrong." The body tells an individual of ill-health in a variety of ways, depending upon the illness: "I jus' feel weak in the legs and then hot and cold" (Leroy's 'flu); "A back ache, and then I get the hot and cold sweats ... When you pass urine, it tends to be a bit stronger than usual" (Earl - any illness); "My nose gets cold and I get a little sniff" (Carlton's cold); "Keep gettin' headaches or feelin' dizzy" (Martha - any illness); and, "Terrible headaches" (Ivy's hypertension). The inability to go to work is also seen to be an early sign of ill-health by most of those who work.

Thus some of the informants appear to have clearly defined ideas about health and illness. Such definitions are, however, more flexible than first appears, depending particularly on the context of any episode of ill-health and on the individual's previous experience. Nevertheless, the definitions that have been expounded above do hold in many cases. Bearing these in mind, it falls upon the next section to consider the informants' ideas on the causes of ill-health in general, and of specific episodes of illness or disease in particular.

The Causes of Ill-Health

Fate

Overall, there is a general acceptance of health and ill-health as part of life, with ill-health being something to be expected and something impossible to prevent. Fatalism runs stongly through many of the interviews, both in connection with health and illness, and life itself. For those who are religious, fatalism is mixed with the power of God's will in determining what will happen to people and why. In many respects, this acceptance of the way things are helps the informants to get on with their lives and to cope with things as they happen. It also means that many of the unpleasant things that happen to them can be faced and dealt with without bitterness or anger.

The young men (Leroy, Earl and Carlton in particular) feel that they have some control over their lives and health: "It's all mapped out for you, your life ... and you've gotta choose the right choices." They choose to improve their health by keeping very fit: "If you look after your body, in the long run, you'll be better off than someone who don't" (Leroy); "I usually keep myself very, very fit, so that if anything comes to me, I'm strong enough not to take any notice of it" (Carlton). The young men also feel, however, that they cannot always influence their health, and that, "Most of the common things that you get disappear within two or three days" (Earl), or that, "If you get an illness, your natural body resistance will get rid of it" (Paul). Fate can, then, play a role: "Legionnaires Disease, for example, you pick that up from a germ, just passing in the air, which is a normal thing. But it could affect one person, and sort of totally miss another. It's a question of fate - who's lucky and who isn't" (Earl). The men, then, hold contradictory ideas. On the one hand, they feel that they can influence their health by keeping fit, but on the other hand, they perceive that some episodes of ill-health just happen because they are determined by fate.

The older women, particularly those with strong religious faith, believe much less in the power of individuals to protect themselves from ill-health. Ill-health is accepted as part of life, against which little can be done: "Whatever you are destined to get, you will get" (Delores); "It's give and take. When it does happen, one should not feel too disappointed. You have to just take it easy and accept it and try to get over it" (Emily); "I break my leg. There was nothin' I could do about that. Yeah! That was jus' somethin' that happen" (Martha). Martha goes on, "I don't worry over sickness. As it comes, you just suffer it. Illness jus' happens, it's nature ... Some people are not healthy, some again, you can't get them sick ... It's just, something natural." Louise also echoes this, "I don't worry about no sickness because what is written is written. Even when I myself became ill, I never moaned, I never grumbled, because we don't buy sickness, it just comes."

All the informants agree that people should expect to be ill sometimes, because, "You're human, innit? You're vulnerable to things" (Carlton). When it does happen, the temptation is always to say, "Why me? But on the other hand, why not you? You are human, and it can happen to you, it can happen to me" (Millie). As Martha indicated, above, some people always seem to be ill, and they seem fated to suffer from ill-health, for reasons that nobody really knows, such as Jean's sister, "the weaklin' of the family", who was, "always bein' ill", and who, "jus' die of natural causes" (Jean).

The fatalism obvious in the conversations about health and illness also emerges in the passages about politics and life in general. As Louise says, "Everything is written for us. That is life." There is consequently a pervasive sense of powerlessness to be able to change thier lives: "I go along with everythin' 'cause there's nothin' you can do" (Ivy); "You cannot change anything" (Jean); "If I was to vote, which I don't usually, 'cause I don't think it's worthwhile, I would vote Labour" (Carlton); and "Power? Me? Aagh!" (Paul). Life, then, is largely out of individual control. The same is true of health, with ill-health an expected and accepted outcome of the "way things are."

Fault

Although fate is the most pervasive influence on the way people think about health and ill-health, the concept of fault also figures in some cases. The idea of individual responsibility for ill-health really acts counter to the influence of fate, but contradictory ideas are quite often held by people, the context being crucial (see, for example, the young men above). The most often mentioned occasion where people are responsible for their health is when they do not take "proper" precautions: "A lot of the time it [ill-health] could be avoided, either pay more attention to all those health warnings and eat the right foods ... a lot of the trouble comes from not taking good advice" (Earl). In a similar way, Delores speaks of people who go out scantily dressed, and then get colds; and Carlton thinks that old people who do not wear hats, often, "bring illness on themselves."

Martha believes that studying too hard will bring on ill-health. Leroy speaks of prostitutes, who, he says, "Have got more chance of catchin' VD than someone like a normal workin' girl." Otherwise, he is not convinced that individuals have any power over their health. In some cases, specific individuals are blamed for their ill-health, although this is rare. Ivy, for example, cannot help but blame her husband for causing his ulcer because, "He was always drinkin', so he didn't have space for eating, or time." Similarly, Carlton blames himself for exacerbating his cold when he played football in the rain. He claims that illnesses are his own fault, "nearly always, but you don't seem to realise it", yet he continues that colds do not seem to follow any sort of pattern of blame. Like most of the informants, he is not really sure, and the context of the illness is crucial to the issue of individual responsibility.

Worries

"Worries" are perceived to be a major cause of ill-health, especially by the older women. Even the younger men can see the importance of worries, particularly Earl, Paul and Danny, whose father, Joe, suffered a severe nervous breakdown fifteen years ago. Joe is a strong believer in the power of worries to make a person ill. He describes his breakdown as, "A terrible headache ... You jus' keep worryin' and feel depressed. You can't really understand what is happening" (Joe). The worries, about some land in Jamaica and his attempts to return there, also had a physical manifestation: an ulcer. Joe thinks that all illnesses are caused by the mind, and that, "If the mind is healthy, I think the body will be healthy"; and consequently, that to overcome ill-health is, "a matter of mind over matters" (Joe).

For the older women, much of their ill-health is perceived to be the result of worries. Ivy, Delores and Ruby all suffer from high blood pressure, Ivy has also been diagnosed as having hypertension, and Ruby has sugar diabetes. As Delores says, "It's your problems that make your body sick - what give you all de aches and pains. You're not relaxed if you've got a problem." Ruby agrees, "If you are worried a lot and have a lot of things on your mind, anythin' will come on you. I was a lot me worried, an' den I was with de sugar [diabetes]." Ivy says, "I have suffered with me hypertension - backward and forward, runnin' from work to work, coping with children. Most of my workmates are black, and we all seem to suffer from this same hypertension." It is here that a link may be made between racism and the women's health. The racism that affects Ruby at work (for full story, see racism section below), she says, "get me upset and depress'. Dat's why we're gettin' blood pressure and sugar ... It get me down, it get me sick, you see, for all dese t'ings bring de sugar up."

Martha also emphasises the importance of worries, especially those that teenagers cause their parents: "That too brings on sickness. Worry do bring on sickness, whatever it is. It's tension and pressure and that, and then your nerves may not be able to take it and then you have a nervous breakdown."

<u>Germs and Viruses</u>

Everybody agrees that some illnesses and diseases are caused by external agents, commonly known as "germs". Their penetrating the body seems to depend a lot upon the strength of individual resistance. Earl says, for example, that germs are, "Here with us all the time, it's just our body resistance goes up and down ... Dependin' on how much you look after your body, your resistance to those germs will fluctuate." Emily recounts the scientific view about the body's resistance: "It is the white blood cells that fight the germs in the body, so if the white blood cells is low, then when the germ gets in the body, it's very difficult to fight it." Martha and Delores do not have this scientific explanation at their disposal, but they agree that the body does resist certain germs. Delores complains that she, "Cannot resist colds, just like your body cannot resist everything." Martha is more philosophical: "Some people's resistance is strong, some people's resistance is low. It depends." When asked on what it depends, Martha replied, "I dunno. Do you?"

The most common germ, or illness caused by a germ, is a cold. Leroy says, "I seem to get a cold once a year. Jus' germs travellin' around in the air." He continues, "This bad 'flu they say comes from Japan. It's in the air, there. You can't help catchin' it" (Leroy). A cold is seen to be an invader of the body, and usually something, "you catch it from one person to another" (Emily). Delores and Carlton, however, conceive of germs as organisms that can penetrate through the skin: "This cold ... gonna rip through my skin" (Carlton); "When you get coughs and colds - that's germs. Especially when they get under the skin, where you can't see it. Then it get sort of bacteria or inflammation" (Delores).

People are seen to be susceptible to germs, just by chance through being in certain places, or because of actions: "I jus' caught it [the 'flu] from a friend or being in the wrong place at the wrong time" (Carlton); "When you finish a game of football and you're really drained, that's when you're susceptible to germs" (Paul). Carlton believes that a high temperature is a good indication of the presence of a germ, "'Cause the body's overheating, like there's something inside the body workin' over time ... something that your body's fightin' against, which isn't too good for you."

The informants are all sure about the existence and effects of germs, because the word is in common usage and they all have experience of "having caught" germs, but they are less convinced of the existence of viruses. Those who have heard of them think they are the same as germs: "Doctors' words, they're all the same as far as I'm concerned. If it's a virus or a this or combination of this and that, they all turn out the same: you're either gonna die of it, or you're gonna live with pain the rest of your life; or it's somethin' they've never heard of that they're jus' puttin' a name to" (Carlton); "They're both germs as far as I'm concerned" (Leroy); "I dunno, I've always thought of them [germs and viruses] as pretty much the same" (Earl); "I went to the doctor and she said it was a virus, but I wanted to ask what a virus is, what she really mean ... I don't like this takin' on of a new word" (Delores).

Heredity

The question of the inheritance of ill-health is not something upon which the informants care to dwell. On the whole, they do believe that some families appear to suffer from certain conditions, and that heredity is quite important, although they do not necessarily feel that this applies to their own families. Delores says, for example, that, "All our troubles might run down to another generation", but as far as her own family is concerned, she says, "I can't say what illness runs, because my father is 77 and he's still workin' on his farm. We have no serious illness in the family what I know of." Similarly, Martha says that, "A disease, that's something ... that can carry on in the family, run on down the generations", but in her family, only good health has been passed down, because her grandmother is still alive and she has several grandchildren herself.

Some of the informants are willing to speculate about which illnesses or diseases may be inherited: "Cancer, that might be passed down through the generations... My Mum's Mum died of cancer, so my Mum could catch it, but I don't like to think about that" (Leroy); "Psoriasis and eczema, they run in the family" (Earl); "Asthma, bronchitis, diabetes [are inheritable]. Sometimes cancer runs in the family, and heart trouble and blood pressure ... [but] sometimes you can see that it skips one generation" (Emily). Ruby also reports that she suffered from asthma all her life, and that it "ran in the family" because an uncle of hers died because of it.

Carlton goes into some detail about the hereditary nature of some conditions, and considers a sex bias in his family: "I know there's a heritage from the father to the son and the son to his son ... I think there's good possibilities of that, 'cause what I've been told about my family past ... there's been a cycle like, especially for the women. The women, they die, they seem to die very early, especially on my mother's side, about 50-55. Like they get something inside them. But for me, for the guys, I think that the guys usually live pretty long in my family." Again, there seems to be the tendency for the informants to see heredity as affecting others, not themselves.

Other Causes of Ill-Health

High on the list of other causes of ill-health comes the environment. This is seen to cause and exacerbate ill-health through the weather, housing conditions, pollution and just by being Britain, rather than anywhere else. These are considered in the Living in Britain section, below. The environment is also seen to be responsible for causing or maintaining germs or colds. Delores, for example, suggests that people often aid the development of a cold by going out inadequately dressed in order to sunbathe, but who then catch a cold when it rains.

Delores has some particularly definite and well-worked out theories about health and illness. She believes, for example, that a lot of the ill-health suffered by women in this country is caused by them failing to use medicines which "clean out" the womb after each period. She bemoans the doctor's lack of faith in preparations such as "Lady Pink" which she used in Barbados: "We know already what creates the sickness and illness in our bodies. That is the womb that we carry ... A good clean out ... That's what we're missin' in this country."

This section on the causes of ill-health is inextricably linked to the other sections, particularly those concerning the effects of living in Britain and the severity of ill-health. Throughout the interviews, instances of episodes of ill-health provoke only occasional guesses at causes, and often the direct cause of the complaint is not known. More important in most cases is the alleviation of the symptoms or effects of the illness or disease, and here cultural factors and fate play leading roles, depending as always upon the context of each case.

The Severity of Ill-Health

Incurable illnesses/diseases

The influence of fate is particularly strong in this category. Some illnesses and diseases are seen to be incurable because they take their fated course, and some will clear up, whereas others will not. Much of the informants' skepticism about the effectiveness of doctors is also present, with conditions such as whooping cough being considered incurable by the techniques of western medicine, although its effects can be ameliorated by the use of traditional remedies such as the taking of a teaspoonful of sugar and grated onion (Ruby and Delores). Earl speaks for everybody when he says that so far he has been healthy and that he would, "like to go out in perfect health, but then I suppose only time will tell."

The men tend to mention specific illnesses or diseases that they are afraid of getting and which they also believe are incurable, such as cancer (Leroy), or cancer, herpes, AIDS and VD (Carlton and Earl). Earl and Carlton are particularly concerned about herpes and AIDS because they have recently read an article about the former's incurability and because the conditions are associated with something they enjoy and do regularly: sex. Carlton confuses the conditions, but is especially afraid of knowing, "that you were gonna die in a space of time." Martha concurs with this view: "I wouldn't like to know if I got cancer or anything like that and that's because there ain't nothin' to do about it." Her religious beliefs, she says, mean that she is not afraid to die.

Almost all of the informants mention cancer at some time as an illness to be afraid of , or one that usually ends in death. Delores, Leroy and Carlton all share the same ideas about cancer, and these are other example of Delores's well worked out theories: "Cancer is a killer. Where it come from? They talk about smoke, but ... my mother die of leukaemia, which'n is a blood cancer - she never smoke ... I honestly think everyone is born with cancer and it jus' takes somethin' to bring it out" (Delores); "Cancer. Everybody's born with it , it jus' takes something to set it off" (Leroy); "Cancer - cancer don't bother me, 'cause cancer is something you jus' gotta fight against ... everybody's got that and it jus' takes something to start it off"

(Carlton).

Delores goes on to challenge a recent medical report that taking the contraceptive pill may lead to higher than average rates of breast cancer. She says, "I can't understand them when they say there's somethin' in the pill that gives you cancer. How can the pill cause the cancer when it's the same, that we all born with cancer, but it jus' takes somethin' to trigger it off?" (Delores). Earl has different ideas about the origins of cancer: "It must be something to do with all these additives they put in food and things they feed to the cows to produce more milk; chickens to produce different coloured eggs ... There's gotta be an answer for that 'cause years ago you didn't hear of cancer."

For the women, the influence of fate and religion are crucial in the case of incurable conditions such as cancer. Martha says, for example, "I goes to church and I believe in God and from my opinion, when things happen, you know, I jus' have to say, 'Well, it happen because it was to happen.' Jus' accept it and forget about it." Similarly, Delores says, "I'm not afraid of gettin' nothin'. Whatever comin' to me, you gotta take it. What's the point of being afraid? Whatever is coming will come to you, so what good is worryin'? Whatever it is, you have to carry it and look to the bible or whatever to help you through it."

The only condition that seems to be viewed as inevitable in old age is rheumatism. Most of the older informants are experiencing or expect to experience pains in the joints which they put down to rheumatism. The younger informants also expect to suffer from it when they get older. The cause of rheumatism is seen to be the cold and damp weather typical of Britain, especially when this is compared with the warm weather of tropical countries. Carlton links rheumatism in the old to chickenpox in the young - both conditions he feels [people] "are bound to have, especially in this country." Martha, Ivy and Delores cannot remember their children having the childhood illnesses such as measles and mumps, although Delores does recall that hers once had chickenpox all at the same time. They do not know why such illnesses should be experienced here and not elsewhere.

Serious illnesses/diseases

When asked if they had had any serious illnesses or diseases, only Martha, Emily and Louise admitted that they had. Martha sufffered from thyroid trouble that was not diagnosed for three years; Emily and Louise both had fibroids and hysterectomies; and Louise also had a mastectomy. Delores, Millie and Ruby have also had hysterectomies, but they did not consider these to be "serious". Delores says, "The only time I was really ill was when I had my hysterectomy"; Millie says that she was, "quite ill", when she had her operation; and Ruby only told of her hysterectomy when she was asked about when she stayed in hospital. The details of their experiences are recorded in the health services section below.

Psychological influences on health

Loneliness is not really something that has bothered any of the informants except Emily. Many of the people who have family and work responsibilities would like the opportunity to be alone sometimes, but they realise that being alone is different from being lonely. Delores, Leroy and Earl feel that loneliness can lead to, "mental illness, not serious illness" (Leroy), and so, "it can make you ill, loneliness can" (Delores). The implication is, however, that they consider mental illness to be less serious than physical illness. Even Emily, who lives alone and has been virtually house-bound for several months after her hysterectomy, does not feel that loneliness is too much of a problem: "Sometimes you feel lonely - take your bible and talk to God! ... Is just another way of talking, and you see that you don't feel lonely."

Tiredness is seen as both a cause of ill-health and as a symptom of it by different informants. Earl recalls that, "Once or twice I've been really run down and get covered in boils and what have you. It's just your body's way of tellin' you that you aren't lookin' after your body properly." Carlton, on the other hand, says, "When I'm really, really tired, I feel that there is something else in my body makin' me feel tired. I don't feel that the illness comes in because I'm tired. If I'm really tired ... then I feel that the illness is there already. That's the cause of what's makin' me tired." Emily agrees, remembering that tiredness was the most obvious symptom of her anaemia.

Delores and Martha believe that tiredness can both cause and be caused by ill-health. Tiredness is a particularly important factor in the women's lives, especially those who work and raise children (Delores, Ivy, Martha, Donna, Judy and Millie). For them, tiredness is a constant companion: "We have the heavy tasks. We rush to get everyone to work, we rush to work, rush at work. Then when you come home, you've got the washin' - set the machine - or cooking, or ironing. It's never ending. Time you finished, you have to go to bed ... Then you get a few hours' rest before you gotta be up again for work ... Tiredness can wear you down" (Delores). Rest can alleviate the tiredness temporarily, but if a person continuously feels tired, Martha suggests that they must be ill.

Most of the informants agree that shock can have effects on health. A sudden shock can cause death, or lead to long-term worries or depression. Emily speaks of some bad news she received which came as a shock and from which it took her a long time to recover. Leroy believes that cancer can be triggered off by shock, but Delores, Martha and Earl feel, like Emily, that it is much more likely to lead on to depression or worries, which they all see as very serious threats to health (see worries section).

Depression can be a serious problem and have effects on health, according to most of the informants. Only two declare that they never get depressed: Louise because of her faith in God, and Millie, who says, "That's one thing I never get." Millie, however, says at another time that she has trouble sleeping because of all the worries about her jobs, health and children, and particularly the health of her son, Ekow, who suffers from sickle-cell anaemia and has to spend quite a lot of time in hospital. The young men admit that they get depressed from time to time, mostly because of worries with money (Paul and Danny), or the threat of unemployment (Carlton and Leroy), or because of thoughts that he could have got a better job (Earl). Donna declares that she only gets depressed when the gas bill arrives.

For the other informants, depression is a much more important factor in their lives. Ruby, for instance, cannot remember a time when she was not depressed. She is depressed by her son who has been gaoled under the "Sus" laws, and about the racial harrassment she claims she is subjected to at work; both of which, she believes, have affected her health directly by raising her blood pressure and causing the development of sugar diabetes. Judy also speaks of being constantly depressed because of worries about her housing conditions, that her children are insecure without their fathers, and that her shift work means that she cannot keep to a routine with her housework, so it always piles up.

The effects of depression on health are thought to be closely related to the effects of worries, and these effects may be substantial (see worries section). Delores says, "You don't eat, make you go skinny, your nerves run down ... it can ruin your health ... All that come from depression." Martha, Emily, Leroy, Carlton and Earl all concur: "Depression is very serious. .. It can lead to mental [illness]" (Emily); "If you worry too much, you can get high blood pressure" (Leroy). Joe also gets depressed sometimes, although not as much as when he had his nervous breakdown. His cure is to read books to try to find out the cause, and then, he says, "It's a matter of mind over matter." The religious people get over their depression through their faith.

Sometimes, some of the informants agree, individuals cannot overcome their depression. Ruby and Judy, for example, cannot see an end to their depression, although Ruby hoped to return to Jamaica, and this she had done before I could interview her for a second time. Joe recalls his breakdown, when he could do nothing to stop it, and his family all report (he does not) that he is still dependent on valium. Carlton speaks with a degree of amazement about how depression changed his personality when he was unemployed: "I used to get vex, especially when it came down to pay days", primarily because he saw others flaunting their pay packets. He continues: "It really gets on my nerves ... You can get yourself to really hate people ... It all goes into your mind, and when you get a job, you realise that is all wrong, it was sending you crazy ... getting depressed" (Carlton).

Thus depression is seen to exacerbate some episodes of ill-health, to cause some others, and also to be an illness in its own right. For some, however, depression is just another "fact of life" to be accepted and overcome as best it can. The next section outlines the ways in which these informants do accept events and cope with them.

Cultural and Personal Inheritance

"Culture" is here loosely defined as those ideas and attitudes which are drawn from a person's heritage and which have some influence on lifestyle and behaviour, and ultimately, their health (see also chapter two).

Remedies

A person's cultural and personal inheritance provides her/him with a set of ways to cope with events (like Schutz's recipes, referred to in chapter four), some of which may be innovative, others of which will be repetitive. Remedies are one such outcome of a person's need to deal with episodes of ill-health, or to overcome discomforts such as headaches or colds.

Only the women from Ghana do not speak at length about the use of remedies, although Millie does mention that her parents used "bush" medicines. Emily may not have had any remedies in her home, or her training as a midwife may have discouraged her from speaking about them.

The younger informants tend to rely on older women for advice about remedies. Donna, Carlton and Leroy rely on Delores; Danny, Paul and Earl use few remedies, but when they do they rely on Joe and Jean; and Judy follows the advice of her friend's mother. Delores, Martha, Ivy, Ruby and Joe have the most to say about remedies, probably because they have had the most experience of them, both in Britain and in the West Indies, and they are able still to get hold of the necessary ingredients or preparations.

During their childhoods, those who were brought up in the West Indies remember that their parents would, "Mix up different bush and make a drink and dat cure you" (Ruby, but echoed by Delores, Ivy, Martha and Joe). For colds, several things were used: "Camphorated oil to rub on the chest and glands" and "ferrol compounds" (Ivy); "black coffee and a squeeze of lemon" (Delores) - with the addition of, "a strong drink, like Bacardi" (Leroy); "ferrol tonic" (Delores); "honey and lemon" (Judy); "peppermint tea, or spice or ginger tea" (Louise, Jean and Joe); and "bayrum" (Danny).

Even the young men prefer to rely on home remedies rather than on drugs from the doctor: "Me mum gave me some home remedies. They was good enough to take everything. I didn't need to go to a doctor" (Carlton). Leroy, Donna and Carlton still use many of the things recommended by Delores, such as olive oil on swellings or rashes because, "It seems to kind of ease it, makes you relax" (Leroy); black coffee with lemon and Bacardi, because, "It keeps your body heated up and that will kill the invading cold in your body" (Carlton); "Alcoholla", for headaches which, "kinda makes your nose tingle, like kinda clears it" (Leroy); and a tonic called "ferrol", which Carlton says, "Helps keep you strong ... It keeps me active."

Earl, a friend of Leroy and Carlton, also uses a strong drink as a remedy for most things: "Jus' wrap yourself up and sweat it out." He also uses herbal teas or hot lemons, and, "after one or two nights of having this treatment, old fashioned remedies", his colds and his children's whooping cough are usually eased. Rubbing rum on the children's chests or giving it to them diluted in a drink also works well, he says. His brothers, Danny and Paul, take mint tea if they feel unwell and they have all tried, "plain dried biscuits with boiled water and ginger tea" (Earl) as a remedy for stomach upsets. Another recipe Earl mentions is "cornflour porridge", which would, "bind your stomach together so you could get away with eatin' a little bit, instead of passin' it all through."

Joe and Jean have an exceptionally large range of home remedies, although Joe admits that, "You cyan't get them very easy here. Some of the time you can get them from the health shops", or from a local "druggist". He speaks of "fever grass", "black mint", ginger and lime, to be made into teas to make you, "sweat it out and be better in no time"; "wintergreen", "sloe linament" and "Canadian stuff" for bites and wasp stings; "bisodol" or "hunters" for his ulcer; and "bitter hollows" for billiousness. Some of these preparations are produced under brand-names.

Ivy speaks of "bayrum", a poultice made of bay leaves, and a popular Jamaican remedy for headaches and feverish feelings; as well as cod-liver oil, "for the bowel system." Martha recommends "cleansing herbs", "For bowels and it regulate the blood ... and cure like what we now call rheumatism, pains." Delores recommends "cod liver malt", which, "clear out your bowels and keeps your system workin'", and she adds, tastes better than cod liver oil. She also speaks of bayrum, grated onion and sugar for whooping cough, and she tells how a nutmeg put in her father's cheek helped him to regain feeling and movement after a stroke. Herbal teas are ubiquitous, being used by all the informants in all the islands represented: Barbados, Jamaica and Dominica.

Specific aspects of the workings of the body, particularly the blood and bowel systems, are the targets for many of the remedies. It can be seen that most of the recipes cause sweating, or "clean out the bowels", or regulate the blood. Delores and Joe have well worked out theories about the blood. Delores says (this is echoed by Martha), "The older you get, your blood gets thinner and you get weaker", and so, by implication, one needs tonics. Joe's theory is quite different from this: "The blood in the body is thicker here than in the Tropics ... I think that cause a lot of this heart disease" (Joe). His theory originates from his mechanical knowledge that, "If you put water through a pump, it will send it through quick", whereas, "with oil, it's much slower ... I jus' draw my own conclusion that if the blood was to run thinner, it wouldn't put a strain on the heart" (Joe).

Joe and Delores do not disagree over the usefulness of tonics. Joe uses "liquid of life", which Danny says, "tastes really horrible." The liquid of life, "is like a wash-out. It clean you", and Joe takes it after a heavy meal. Ferrol is used as a tonic by Leroy and Ivy, not just to keep colds away, but, "to keep everythin' goin'" (Ivy). Ganga (or marijuana) also serves as a tonic, whether smoked, or used as a tea or mixed with rum in the traditional fashion. Ruby takes "Strongback", which is made from seaweed and, "tastes bittery, like de woods back 'ome." More western preparations such as Wincarnis, Sanatogen and iron tablets are also used (Judy and Delores).

Two of the young men have devised tonics of their own, with a little help from Delores and Jean. Leroy's recipe consists of, "raw egg with milk mixed in with sugar and nutmeg", which he says makes him feel very good, very strong. Earl's recipe consists of, "Guinness with raw egg, grated carrots - squeeze the juice out of the carrots - and a bit of nutmeg", which fills him up and contains, he says, good things like iron.

Most of those who mention using remedies also say that they prefer to try their own remedies first, before they will even consider seeing a doctor. If, after a period of three days, the complaint has not disappeared, then they will usually visit a doctor. For unexpected or unusual conditions, a doctor may be consulted while a remedy is also employed. The attitude of using doctors as a last resort is also reflected in the attitude to drugs, most of which are disliked.

Most of the remedies and recipes referred to above are in a liquid form and almost all the informants believe that liquid medicines are superior to tablets or pills. Some will take pills if there is no alternative: "I will only take a tablet if I'm really bad, bad, bad, bad, bad, bad! ... Don't like puttin' them down my system ... They take me outa my way of doin', my scene ... I'd rather trust something from me mum than from a doctor, even if I was dyin'" (Carlton, but echoed by many others). Paul is one of the few to say that pills work at all, and he only says this because he has recently taken some that cleared up his stomach-ache. Danny thinks that tablets are all placebos: "Most of the time it's kidology. You know, a few coloured tablets and your brain does the rest"; and Earl prefers to do without anything: "With or without the drugs doesn't make any difference." Donna also prefers to let illness "pass" without taking drugs.

Over and over again, some of the informants air their views about the efficacy of, and their preference for, liquid medicines and home remedies: "Medicine is better than when they give you tablet " (Louise); "Medicines - liquid. That's the best ... we're not used to pills" (Martha); "I think the medicine is better than the pill" (Donna); "I don't like tablets ... I like medicine, liquid, and I would go for the 'ome remedy" (Delores); "Back 'ome dey give you medicine, not pills. <u>Real</u> medicine. The medicine wash out your insides ... I cyan't take capsule - it make me sick ... You feel the medicine workin' more than you feel the pills" (Ruby).

The reasons for this preference for liquids are many. Most obvious is that home remedies are liquids and some of these are known to work. Louise says that pills are addictive, whereas liquids are not. Martha just says, "it's what we're used to - it's not necessarily better." Ruby genuinely feels that medicines work better, that they act as a wash-out, and can be felt to be working. Similarly, Delores says, "Whatever sickness you get, it is in the blood. What water would do, where water would wash, a tablet cyan't do ... A tablet have to dissolve before it can do de trick, but if you take a glass of medicine, it mean it go through the body. If you're lyin' down, you can feel it." Earl adds that, "At least in liquid form, you can see some form of whatever you're takin'. In tablet form, it could be anything."

Paul, Leroy, Emily and Delores all say that they do not like any drugs, and would always prefer to, "live natural" (Emily). All of these attitudes to drugs are of crucial importance, and may help to explain the often raised issue of non-compliance. Most of these informants do not believe in the power of western drugs, paticularly pills, and many of them do not take their prescribed doses (see health services section). In the majority of episodes of ill-health, home remedies are used and are effective, and this represents a large benefit from their cultural, family and personal heritages. The degree of reliance on these preparations is huge, and yet this is a neglected area of study. Earl and Joe in particular bemoan the ignorance of their doctors and see it as a real waste, because the making of remedies is becoming, "a dyin' art" (Earl). Joe is also worried about the chemicals from which drugs are made, and thinks that researchers should turn their interest to the medicines of the third world, made from natural ingredients.

Religion

Seven of the informants attend a place of worship regularly: Delores, Ruby and Donna go to a spiritualist church, the New Testament Church of God; Ivy goes to a Pentecostal church; Martha to an Anglican one; Emily to the Divine Prayer Society; and Louise to a church she refers to as "Christian" (ie Evangelical). Of the others, four are keen to declare that they are religious, but do not attend church for a variety of reasons: Millie sends her children, but has not got the time to go herself; Leroy says he has not got the time; Joe says, "It's not like back home ... I like to be felt wanted in a place, and it doesn't feel good if the people who're comin' there are all strangers"; and Carlton feels that, "You don't have to go to a church to believe in Jesus Christ."

Danny, Paul and Earl say that they used to go to church when they were children, but, "As you get older, you become more broad minded" (Danny), and, "You get out of the routine" (Earl). Judy is the only one who did not express some religious beliefs, even from her childhood.

On the whole, the younger people are much less passionate about and convinced of their religious beliefs, and several are openly skeptical about the value of religion. Leroy believes that religion can help some people, like his mother and people of her generation: "It helps them to carry on ... a little pray, and she comes out relaxed", but he does not think it is necessary for him. Earl feels that it does not make, "a great deal of difference healthwise", but that it can help, "mentally, because ... believin' in something can help you over certain emotional problems which can be beneficial to your health." They feel, then, that religion can help with non-physical complaints. Carlton is the most openly hostile. He accepts that his mother wants to go to church, and that it can help her psychologically, but he also believes that, "There's some people in there, people who are not believers ... [and] I'm sure, I'm positive sure, it was somebody done something to her ... I'm sure they put something in her eye ... 'cause she went to that church perfect one day; next day she woke up, next day, she couldn't <u>see</u>" (Carlton). Delores, however, thinks conditions at work were to blame for her eye infection and temporary blindness.

For most of the women, however, religion is an extremely important force in their lives, and one that links up with other important factors such as racism and fate. On the whole, the religious women see religion as a comfort, a giver of strength and a diffuser of any anger they feel against the way things are. Hence it helps them to overcome episodes of ill-health and racial dicsrimination. For some, religion also has a direct beneficial effect on health, either through the healing churches or through its calming, accepting influences. All through the interviews with Ruby, Delores, Ivy, Martha, Emily and Louise in particular, the power and pervasiveness of religion comes through.

Louise's faith controls her whole life, and allows her to feel peaceful and to gain strength. It has helped her overcome her two serious operations almost without worry: "I never cry, jus' call on Him, because He is there to help me in all my needs. I have faith in God, I don't take tablets. God is always there with me, to heal me ... When I go for the op., God always revives me quick. I cannot complain." Louise accepts everything that happens to her without qualms or complaints, just relying on a combination of God and fate to control her life.

Religious beliefs clearly help to alleviate the worries that could be caused by everyday life and lead on, in turn, to ill-health (see worries section). As Emily says, "It is very important to have God in your life ... because, you see, a lot of heavy burden is taken off your shoulders because you know that what is worryin' you, you have poured everything out to Him." For Ivy, her faith can block out the unpleasantness of everyday life: "My great enjoyment is goin' to church ... I can go into church for half and hour, and then when I go home, I feel quite refreshed, peaceful, and I forget all the aggro at work, and I think about the scripture and the powers."

This is true also for Ruby, who is depressed almost continuously about conditions at work and her son's future. She says, "Is only the Almighty God you must put your trust to. I leave everything in his hands ... I don't trust in men, only in God ... I'm prayin' to God. It give me strength to work another coupla years and then go home." She recalls that the Race Relations Board, called in by Delores and herself to deal with the matron at work, wanted her permission to prosecute, but she refused, saying, "No. God will do the work for me." Consequently, the matron continued to oppress the black workers, and Ruby and Delores have continued their passive resistance, strengthened by their faith.

Delores and Ruby attend healing churches, and their skepticism of the NHS and western medicine means that in many cases, they prefer to use the healing services and their own remedies rather than GPs. Delores describes what goes on: "We see a lot of people come there sick, stroke, can't walk ... What we use is olive oil, massage that oil, prayin' water, we pray, and the one who can see, whom God raised to do that, him massage 'em ... And dat do de trick." Ruby concurs, "If you sick, them pray for you, heal you and you get better. Is only the Almighty God you must put your trust to."

Faith can also help in specific cases: "I got all the doctors confused, that how come I could walk around with a hb of six [the normal haemoglobin level in the blood is twelve or thirteen] - I say, well, I'm walking with God" (Emily). Delores believes that faith and health are inextricably linked: "If you haven't got faith in God, then you will make the whole body ill ... the moment you sit down and say, 'Look, I can't go on any more', then you become <u>ill</u>."

For some of the informants, then, the reliance on religion is total, to help them to cope with, and get through, everyday experiences, including episodes of ill-health. For many of the others, religious beliefs are very important and mesh with the power of fate in controlling their lives and determining their reactions to, or more commonly acceptance of, events and occurrences in everyday life. Faith not only outlines the ways to cope with events and worries, but also gives strength and peacefulness to overcome difficulties, often through acceptance or passive resistance. The influences specifically on health are enormous for some of the informants, particularly those who attend healing churches, but also for others whose faith in God usually far outstrips their faith in physicians. Thus religious beliefs help the informants psychologically, and alleviate psychosomatic conditions as well as giving them the strength to overcome physical complaints.

<u>Food</u>

All the informants believe that food has an important role in the maintenance of good health. For some it is the correct balance of foods that is beneficial; for others it is the need for specific sorts of foods. For some of those who have spent a large proportion of their lives abroad, the food they can obtain here is compared with their memories of what food was like abroad, and rarely is the food in Britain preferred. Again there are differences between the younger and older informants, the younger being more acquainted with westernised foods and some of them preferring these; and the older tending to prefer the traditional food they remember from their childhoods. Direct links are made between foods and health or ill-health in many cases.

The idea of a mixture of foods, or a good balance is important to some. Earl suggests, "a balance of vegetables. The meats, they're not so important, but it's the vitamins, proteins, natural fibres." Joe feels that balance is especially needed in this country: "Eating a proper meal or diet, I think that is very important, especially with us coloured people. Comin' here, we're changin' a long-time pattern." This is an acute problem for Joe because he has an ulcer, but cannot eat at regular times because his shifts change from week to week.

Martha is another advocate of a mixture of food: "If you balance your food, it's all right. Bit of this, bit of that. Plenty of greens, and jus' balance the starches ... If you always stick to a balanced diet, I think your health will be all right." Emily concurs, but at the time of the life-story interview, she did not have a working cooker and so was eating a very poor diet.

Many of the informants stress the importance of eating some foods and avoiding others. Jean says, "It depends on what food you gonna eat. If you're gonna stuff yourself with fatty food and sweet things, you might as well don't bother." She advocates eating fresh greens, and grilling or roasting meat to reduce its fat content. Earl agrees, and points out that sweet and sticky things are especially bad, and he complains about the additives they put in western food. Martha feels that starchy food is, "Not good for your blood ... I don't eat much of our food such as sweet potatoes, yams, plantains."

The preference of many of the informants for traditional food is, however, striking. The younger men and women tend to eat a mixture of western "junk" food and traditional food. Danny, Paul and Judy prefer what they call "conventional" food, such as sausage and chips. Earl and Carlton, however, prefer the West Indian food their mother prepares. Earl feels nostalgic about the past: "I dunno whether it was the way it was cooked or where she [mother] got it from, but it seemed to be makin' you grow all the time. You was that much fitter." Carlton gives a long defence of his preference for traditional food, which includes: "Tradition. West Indian food, I take it as the strongest part of my livin'." He goes on to tell that his ability to run fast comes directly from the food that he eats.

The freshness of traditional West Indian food in the West Indies is something preferred by many of the informants, and they feel it has important effects on health. They remember: "The food was fresh, so that what build your health, and das why, where I come from, we didn't have to see much doctor" (Delores); "If you buy the meat, it should've jus' come from de goat, pig or cow ... Dat is <u>fresh</u>" (Ruby); "If you want a bit of steak, it would be freshly killed" (Joe); and, "It was a hot climate, you ate <u>fresh</u> food. Nothin' is stored" (Carlton).

On the other hand, the food in Britain is disliked: "A lot of the food you get now from the supermarket is junk food - monosodium glutamate" (Earl); "This place is jus' things in tins and they're stale or frozen" (Carlton); "Since I come here and you eat, and you don't have no healt' for the food is not fresh" (Ruby). The dislike of frozen food is particularly strong among a few: "We eat too much ice. The meat, it takes away all the "vrershen" [dialect word for variety and strength]. We eat dat. Dat is trash ...All the nourishments is all gone into the ice. Ice draws it out ... If I make things, I like 'em natural" (Delores); "We haffi get de frozen meat and heat it and so dat's why we don't have our healt'" (Ruby); "The food here is fridged, frozen. It is not fresh. All this food is no good. We eatin' it. All right, it won't kill us, but the <u>fresh</u> food is best" (Louise). Carlton and Joe also complain about frozen food.

Some foods are seen to be important when people are suffering from ill-health. Following on from the preference for liquid medicines (see remedies section), several of the informants stress the need for liquids when a person feels unwell. Earl says, "If you're like seriously ill, take plenty of fluids." He is echoed by Carlton, Leroy, Emily and Delores, who says that all that is necessary when one is ill, "is nourishin' things like liquids, like soup, fluids, as much as you can" (Delores). Earl and Leroy also have their tonics to keep them healthy (see remedies section). Lack of food is implicated by Ivy in causing her husband's ulcer, and Judy believes that her son's reluctance to eat is the cause of his susceptibility to colds and throat infections.

Thus, as most would agree, "I think it [food] have a lot to do with de healt', an' it keep you fit" (Joe). It is important to remember also that many of the home remedies are based on many of these ideas about food, and that they are largely composed of different sorts of foods and drinks (see remedies section). Foods and drinks are seen to be one of the few ways in which health can be improved or maintained. They may also be a major beneficial element of a person's cultural heritage, allowing a wide range of choice.

Temperature and "Hot and Cold"

The importance of temperature is linked with the need to have balance in the body. A "normal" temperature signals health, and any deviation from this is seen to be indicative of some sort of ill-health. Carlton, for example, when he feels that he has a cold, takes black coffee, lemon and a strong drink to, "keep my temperature normal." Earl and Leroy emphasise the importance of being, "the right temperature", otherwise, "you might have 'flu" (Leroy). Earl has some sort of grading system, for he says he always checks his children's temperatures when they feel unwell, to see, "whether they are just a bit flushed or hot, or whether they are actually ill."

A high temperature seems to be immediately indicative of ill-health: "I look all right, but if you take the temperature and find it is above, so then you know that I am sick" (Delores); "Get the temperature ... That means the body tellin' you there is something wrong" (Emily); "Your temperature is a lot to do with your health, because'n if your temperature shot up, somethin' wrong; if it's too low, something's wrong" (Martha); and a temperature, "automatically tells me I am sick, 'cause my body's overheating" (Carlton).

Temperature, then, is an important sign of ill-health. The question of the broader importance of the concepts "hot and cold", however, do not mean anything to these informants of Afro-Caribbean descent. Questions in the focused talk arose from some answers given by some of the Asian informants in the life-story interviews (see chapter six), but were asked of this group to check whether or not they were specific to any group.

Miscellaneous factors

With all the modern health education material on the issue of weight, I thought it important to ask the informants whether or not they thought weight could affect health. Several of the people interviewed could be considered overweight, especially Ruby, Delores, Martha, Jean and Emily. The informants' views on the issue of weight are varied and sometimes contradictory - perhaps representing a clash between "traditional" views and modern propaganda.

Millie, Donna and Judy are the only ones who are really concerned about their weight. They all want to be thin, but like food too much to be able to keep on the diets they go on. The young men also want to be slim, but they also want muscle, and so advocate doing plenty of exercise. Earl and Leroy can see only advantages in being slim and disadvantages in being fat: "A fat person's gotta do more work ... puttin' more strain on his heart and blood vessels" (Earl); "Fat people got more risk of dyin' of heart attacks than slim people" (Leroy). Carlton, however, can see both advantages and disadvantages in being fat: "Skinny people, I think are the healthier", but he adds that he rarely sees fat people in doctors' surgeries, so, "they've got a lot of flesh on them, so the cold's got more to penetrate through."

The women who are overweight are not at all convinced that weight can have any serious effects on health. Some of them say that they have big bones and have always been big, and it annoys them that their doctors want them to lose weight (Ruby, Martha, Delores, Ivy and Emily). Emily, who is the largest, says: "They say the slim person is healthier because they carry less weight - that is true, but then again, some people can be slim and they are not well ... and you can get some plump or solid and they are all right ... So, it depends. If a person has been healthy all their lives, they should be OK." Martha agrees, "Some people born to be fat and they're healthy, and some people thin and they're healthy."

This lack of agreement with "official" or medical opinion is also evident in their discussions about smoking. Seven smoke cigarettes regularly, one smokes them occasionally, one smokes a pipe, and seven do not smoke at all. Nine of the informants are not convinced that smoking can be bad for health, because of their own experiences. Ruby, who used to smoke a pipe, says, "Some people don't smoke and still have bad healt', so dat mean de smokin' don't doin' no damage to nobody's healt'." Jean, Donna and Judy, who are all regular smokers enjoy the habit; Jean is a social smoker, and Donna and Judy smoke to keep their weight down. Martha and Emily, who do not smoke, are unsure of the dangers of smoking because they do not smoke. Joe has mixed feelings: he smokes a pipe and says, "I don't believe smokin' is bad for you ... My grandma, she always smoke a clay pipe and she live until 109 ... What is <u>bad</u> for de healt' is de chemicals dat go into the tobacco. That's why I gave up smokin' cigarettes."

Earl, who smokes regularly, and Delores, who smokes occasionally, think that there are clear benefits to health from smoking, particularly smoking marijuana: "I smoke a cigarette or marijuana to soothe. It keep me calm, comfort me ... I don't say it's bad for your health because some people that don't smoke suffer with bad health in different ways ... Some say it give you cancer, but my mother never smoked and she died of cancer. We don't know what's ruinin' our health" (Delores); and Earl concurs: "I smoke cigarettes or hash or marijuana from time to time ... it helps you, thought-wise, I think. It seems to open up your mind, relax you", but he also concedes that smoking is, "what brought the bronchitis back."

Very few of the informants are totally convinced that smoking is bad for health, and if they do, it is related to their own experience: "When people smoke, you can see the smoke that is on their fingers. How that goin' to affect the inside of your heart?" (Louise, echoed by Ivy); and, "Inhalin' tar and things, and some of the stuff lines the lungs and it's got to go black or cause something eventually" (Paul). Only Leroy mentions the most heavily publicised outcome of smoking: "As you get older, it's bad and you might get lung cancer." Leroy, Carlton, Danny and Donna intend to give up "soon" because of its feared effects, and because it hampers the younger men in sports.

Sport and exercise are very important to a number of the informants, and most believe that exercise is good for health. Even Jean, who is 58 years old, insists, "If I get the chance, I'm on the floor, doin' a coupla press-ups!" Exercise is seen to be good because it keeps the body fit and reduces the fat (Delores and Judy), and tones up the muscles (Donna). Several of the women think that exercise is good, but cannot do much themselves, either because they have not got the time (Martha, Ruby, Ivy), or because they lack basic fitness (Louise, Emily). Joe thinks that exercise is essential in Britain because, "You don't perspire half as lot as in the Tropics ... You don't have to do special exercise in the Tropics to keep fit or feel fit, 'cause jus' by walkin' ... you'd be perspirin' and it trims you and makes you feel fresh and fit."

For the younger men, exercise is exceptionally important. Leroy and Earl feel that they get sufficient exercise at work, although Leroy, with Carlton, Danny and Paul, all do exercise in their leisure time, training and/or playing football. They all believe that exercise does them good: "You feel a lot better, you spring out of bed, you're more alive" (Paul); "You can prolong your life a bit" (Danny); "You gotta keep your body in good condition ... or your joints will jus' weaken up" (Carlton); "It's very important to keep your body in good shape ... If you look after your body, I think in the long run, you'll be better off than someone who don't" (Leroy).

Thus things such as exercise and good food can help the body defend itself against ill-health, but they cannot actually prevent the onset of illness or disease, which is more or less determined by fate and/or God's will. Traditional remedies represent a particular and specific way of coping will ill-health, and they offer a necessary alternative to doctors practising western medicine who are viewed typically with suspicion and skepticism. Health education information about smoking, weight and the value of frozen foods, is not easily accepted by people whose cultural beliefs suggest the opposite, and often it seems that only personal experience can overthrow deeply held beliefs, as, for example, Earl, who believes that smoking can have beneficial effects "thought-wise", but who also feels that it is responsible for his bronchitis.

Living in Britain

Racism

Only two informants say that they have had no experience of racism in Britain. For some, racism is a pervasive force: "It is there and you know it's there. You can feel it all the time, everywhere. You know you're black" (Ivy); "It's always that all these years" (Delores); "It happens so often that you can't be bothered to argue with people any more" (Emily); "Some are prejudiced and they might chuck you out. There's a lot of that racial stuff ... there's a lot of things that happen 'cause of your colour" (Leroy).

Others report specific incidents of racism that upset them. The women who work at the old people's home, for example, all speak of the matron, whom, they claim, is an avowed racist. Ruby has been particularly affected, because it is she who is picked on, and who was sacked when she went to Jamaica to bury her mother. Ruby believes that the pressure put on her by the matron has directly caused her ill-health, and the ill-health of her work-mates: "All these things doin' to us in there ... That's why some of them in there have blood pressure, some are sugar [have sugar diabetes]" (Ruby). She says that when the matron picks on her, she feels, "de sugar rise up. Is what she have done to me have cause me to have dis sugar, for I worry a lot" (Ruby), and on one occasion, "I get <u>HOT</u>. De sugar must've rise up in me ... I was, gone! I was tremblin' all over" (Ruby). After this incident, Ruby was off work for four weeks with anxiety state and depression.

It is not only Ruby who reports the effects of the matron's racism. Ivy says, "She makes it obvious she doesn't like blacks. She show it." Delores, a close friend of Ruby's, shares some of her difficulties: "I try to work with Mrs White [the matron]. We are all people, not colour, <u>PEOPLE</u> ... She chuck out Ruby ... I put the union on to it. Mrs White say, 'I don't know why the Council employs these blacks, I'm goin' to split them up'" (Delores). Millie says, "She doesn't like black people"; and Judy that, "The atmosphere there is wrong. At that home, they separate the blacks and whites [workers] onto two different floors - the difficult ones [old people] downstairs who can't do nothin' for themselves, and the blacks get put there."

It is not only these women who have experienced racism at work. Several of the men say that most of the discrimination that they have noticed has occurred at work. Earl remembers that when he was unemployed, he applied for thirty or forty jobs and in the interviews he had there would be several whites, and although he was convinced that he had better qualifications and presented himself better, he would always be turned down. Paul says that people often react to him at work: "There are times when you can <u>tell</u> they're gonna say something to you, or look at you like that and say, 'Oh! he's not like he should be - not a text-book type, he's not what I imagined.' That's the case lots of times."

Leroy and Carlton have experienced racism at work too. Leroy recalls, "I went to school to get better qualified and they wasn't payin' me. The guy I went to school with, who's white, they did [pay]." Carlton found a job as a play worker, but eventually discovered that he was the only black employee because he could control the , "bad, bad kids that would beat up the babies." Any applications by other blacks were rejected even after interviews when Carlton was present and thought the person suitable. He also wonders about the banks: "The bank people, they wouldn't give me a decent loan. I dunno whether it's because of my colour, but I know lots of coloured guys who've tried to get loans and failed" (Carlton). Emily has also experienced discrimination at work: "If I have a job to do, I do it in the same way as a white person would do, but if my work is not accepted, it's not something for me to bother my head about because I know that I have done what I know is good."

Although many of the informants try to shrug off racism, probably because it is accepted to be just part of life, it does affect some of them deeply. Donna, for example, gave a powerful nine-minute speech after a question on racism, including such things as: "The government ... they would like the black people to leave ... They wanted people to come and do all the dirty jobs, sweep the roads and so on, run the buses - all the jobs the people here didn't want to do. Now that these people have worked over here, had their children here, why should they be made to leave? Especially if they don't want to go ... They've put their labour into this country. I'll never think of this country as <u>my</u>

country ... but I think it's unfair that people who've made their lives here, worked ... to then be forced out of the country... Some people, like mostly a lot of English people, they can't accept the country's been "invaded" [ironic tone] by Indians, blacks, Greeks and that. They don't like it. Me, I'm not bothered ... I'd be really annoyed if someone said to me, 'Go back to your own country.' I mean, I don't class this as my country, but it's where I've lived since I was seven..."

"In certain countries what is black countries like South Africa, Australia, and now English people have taken over, and you don't hear an uproar about that ... nobody's really breakin' down barriers about that, to say, well, that was a black man's country, and now white people have taken over ... In certain countries, black people are not allowed to go and yet it's their country, but run by a white government and what can you do? You can say all these things, but people don't understand - 'We just want you out of England', you know ... There's a lot of people in England think that, but I jus' don't let them bother me. I'm just here to work for myself and I don't care what you think - nothing you say is goin' to depress me" (Donna).

Carlton is very pessimistic about the future in Britain because of racism: "I'm not goin' somewhere jus' because of my colour, I'm goin' as an individual ... It's gotta stop somehow. Like unless you stop it, it ain't gonna stop. Then people will jus' fight fire with fire; people will get mash up. You can't stop. Once something's started that's bad, you can only treat it with bad. It has to get worse before it gets better. It's gettin' worse." As Carlton points out, "This body, it's jus' the outside of my inside. I jus' lookin' through this skin. What matters is inside."

Martha and Delores are paticularly insistent that there should be no discrimination between the races, as it was, they say, in Barbados. Martha says, "In my country, I was brought up with white people. My mother was a domestic servant, and I was brought up with the children, altogether. So, to me, I don't see no difference. Some people are different, but if you brought up that way, it don't worry you. You pity them." Delores emphasises the effect racism can have on black people: "I don't even like to think what the effect is. It can wear people down ... It makes you feel bad inside, angry, and then one day it will come out ... This racial thing, we will get over it. We have to live through it and be strong. We have to. It's the only way to carry on, to survive" (Delores).

There are other instances that offend the respondents. Earl, for example, says that because his girlfriend is white, when they go out he is often looked at as if, "what's that black so-and-so doin' with her." On a couple of occasions, he says they have been met by aggressive individuals, shouting abuse, and in one case, something was thrown at them out of a car, along with the usual abuse. Danny remembers that he could not get into West End clubs because they did not want to admit blacks. Leroy speaks of the attitudes at school: "My mates, even ... they used to pick on me ... I don't know why we have to go through this, bein' shown up. It gets me mad."

It is Delores, however, who delivers the most forthright and the longest speech about racism. She spoke for some twenty minutes, having been sparked off by the question, "How are things at work, these days?" She begins by recounting the question of a man from head office who came to investigate the allegations of racial harrassment at her workplace: "Him from Head Office, he say to me, 'Which country are you from?' I told him that we are one, that his father is my father who is our creator ... He ask me, 'Where you come from?' I say, 'Small England.' He say, 'Where's that?' I say, 'Don't you know? You see, you all don't travel ... You don't read your history. If you did, you wouldn't have no hatred in your hearts for anybody, not blacks, Indians, nobody. You all think the blacks don't know history. We went to school. You got it that we come outa the jungle, but if you get on a plane and go to Barbados, you will see that it is no jungle ... Barbados is jus' like here, only small. You got jungle here? No, right. Africa got jungle, yeah! But the white man - that is the English-man - go to Africa and take over and <u>put</u> the blacks in the jungle' ... As small as my country was and is, this is the mother country. She comes and she takes everything and what she gonna buy from our country, you gotta sell for next to <u>nothin'</u> because she's the <u>mother</u> ... I say, 'So my mother gotta feed me! I'm here to be fed. I'm here to drink milk and honey until I ready to go back and you're not gonna send me back' ... Because of my colour, why should people treat me as - what - rubbish?" (Delores).

Delores concludes with the idea that people who let themselves worry about racism could, "worry to death." All those who have experienced racial dicrimination believe that it can have effects, because of racial attacks and because it leads to fights and worry. Ruby links racism directly to her own ill-health, and she also believes that the large proportion of blacks who suffer from high blood pressure and/or hypertension is another direct result of racism. The effects, mental and physical, may, therefore, be enormous.

Work

Work is an important factor in the lives of all those who are working. Only two of the informants were not working at the time of the first interview: Emily used to be a midwife, but left work when she became ill with anaemia, and she has not worked since; and Louise used to work in a factory, but has not been able to work since the first of her two major operations. Carlton was out of work when he was asked the focused questions, having been made redundant from his job mixing chemicals in a record manufacturing factory. All of those not working wish they were. Louise says, for example, "When I was workin', I was very happy, because when you get up in the morning, you clock your card in, and then on a Friday, you have a bit of money. Now I have to wait on Social Security to give me a penny on which to live."

Carlton is particularly angry and upset that he is not working. He had a period of unemployment before he got his last job, and he remembers it as a time of great depression and worry: "The whole incentive to do anything was gone ... You have so much in you, if someone was to come at me at the wrong moment, I'm sure I'd just rip their head off their shoulders with my bare hands, you know? The pressure inside jus' fill me up ... I think I was going mad. I used to talk to myself" (Carlton). In the final interview, unemployed again, he desperately wants another job.

Most of the informants worry about unemployment. Earl half-jokes that it could cause you to, "starve to death", and he feels that the worry of it all, "must play a big part in people's health." Danny worries about his prospects because he has seen many of his fellow workers being put on short-time or being made redundant. Leroy feels that, "If I lost my job, that would really crack me up ... My work is very important." None of the women wants to lose her job either: "If I stayed at home it would affect my health because I would be bored, stiff bored" (Jean).

As indicated at the beginning of this chapter, five of the informants work in the same old people's home in north London: Ruby, Delores and Ivy work as full-time care assistants, Millie as a laundry worker during the day and as an office cleaner at night, and Judy as a temporary care assistant. Jean works as a canteen assistant and a tea lady; Martha is a cleaner in a place she could only name "off the record" during the day, and as a supervisor in a youth club in the evenings; Donna is a clerical worker in a local electricity showroom; Joe is a fitter, working shifts for British Rail; Earl is a maintenance engineer in a West End hotel; Leroy is a scaffolder; Paul an insurance clerk; Danny a toolmaker; and Carlton used to work in a factory.

All of those working like their jobs, although several work in difficult, sometimes dangerous conditions, and some believe that their work could have severe effects on their health. Others, however, feel that their work has beneficial effects. Leroy, for instance, says that being a scaffolder is good for him: "You get fresh air, you're movin' about all the time. Since I been there, I feel I'm a bit stronger .. I think it's doin' me good." This is despite the several injuries he has received: a groin strain which he is worried about: "Once it's there, it might never go away. It's a weakness that won't go away ... I can still feel it, like a lump." He also has a lump on his wrist, which he says is "displaced gristle". Donna, Martha and Jean are the others who feel that their work can have no ill effects on their health.

The women who work at the old people's home share fears about the effects it must have on their health. They all work long hours and shifts, but they all say they enjoy their work and like to care for the old people even though, "those old people we care for call us black bastards" (Delores). They all agree with Delores when she says, "although it might not be good for the health, I enjoy doin' it."

Ivy, Ruby and Delores all tell of accidents at work that have resulted in severe shoulder, back and knee injuries, caused usually by slipping or tripping on the stairs or floors, or through lifting "stroppy" residents. Delores and Judy also report that they have had eye infections which they believe are caused by the acidy urine of the old people. Ruby says, "the work we doin' affect you, make you sick." Judy goes on, "[the residents] are really smelly, like the ones that suffer from cancer and Parkinson's. You've got all sorts of things coming out of them and you've gotta inhale that when you're changin' them ... Sometimes you can feel it breathin' down you." Millie washes the linen, and says, "everythin' you washin' is terrible smellin'. Even though there is no infection there, you can still get something."

As indicated in the racism section, Ruby feels strongly that the conditions at work, and particularly the attitude of the matron, are directly linked to her high blood pressure and sugar diabetes. Tiredness is also a pervasive problem for her, Delores and especially Millie who has to go home after work, cook for her children, and then go out again to do an evening job because she needs the money.

Chemicals in the workplace were seen to be threats to the health of Louise and Carlton. Louise used to work in a factory, and when asked if she thought the work could have affected her health, she says, "I thought it did, at the time. We used to work a lot with chemicals - hairsprays, powders, sun lotions and stuff ... I worked there eight and a half years, and from then on I was sick" (Louise). Her cancer was diagnosed while she was working there. Carlton also worked with chemicals, and said, when he worked there, "I know there's things in that place could kill me, or do me harm. I'm not too sure about permanent damage, but I'm sure this could give you damage for years ahead and it can get into your body, and if you have children, I know they can come out not how they're supposed to be."

Joe and Danny also work in dangerous environments. Joe complains first about his irregular shifts which mean that his digestive system never settles down and gets set in a pattern. He fixes diesel trains and says of the fumes, "Although we have extractor fans, you can actually taste it, feel it goin' onto your chest." To overcome this, he drinks, "hot chocolate. It's known that if you work in a lot of paint, you should drink a lot of milk - it wash out the lungs straight away" (Joe). He also thinks there is a problem with asbestos: "They didn't worry about asbestos ten years ago ... Now they give us a cotton mask ... That asbestos is dangerous, 'cause it can't burn, it jus' powder up and you might breathe all that in and it stick to your lungs inside and it must affect you."

Despite his specific fears, Joe enjoys his work and wants to be fit enough to carry on. So far, he has passed all the necessary medicals. Danny feels the same. He worries about the dust from grinders he uses, "Which cause silicosis, like miners get, and it slowly kills you"; the glare from welding torches, and flying metal which has cut him on many occasions. He adds that the firm he works for cannot afford to follow all the safety precautions because if it did it would go out of business. Danny is worried about this, but accepts it as, "the name of the game."

Earl and Paul worry about the confined spaces in which they work. Paul feels that working in an overcrowded office means that he is exposed to too many colds. Earl says that flourescent lights give him, "headaches, general sort of nausea feeling", and he adds that the visitors to the hotel often bring with them new strains of germs which he is consequently exposed to.

Thus the informants have a very sensitive concern for the effects that their working conditions can have on their health, but, in general, they accept these conditions as being "part of the job". Almost all of them enjoy working and fear the prospect of unemployment much more than the possible injuries to their health. In many cases, their definition of health is closely tied to their work: to be healthy is to be able to work. To be ill, consequently, is usually defined as being unable to work. These echoes of Parsons' theory of the sick role are taken up in chapter seven.

The Environment

The environment of Britain is thought by the informants to affect their health through the weather, housing conditions and racial discrimination. The case of racial discrimination has been discussed above. The weather and housing conditions are seen to be a cause of ill-health when compared with conditions as they are remembered elsewhere. Some of the informants base their answers on their own experience; others give opinions on imagined cases.

Earl believes that cleanliness is the most important factor: "If you're livin' in a fairly clean environment, you are not gonna get as affected as someone workin' in a sewer or a lavatory. It must be quite important in determining how your health goes." Leroy agrees, mentioning London specifically: "Livin' in London! If you were out in the country, you'd breathe all the fresh air and all that lot. It might not matter a great deal, but livin' in this sort of area with all these cars and chimneys and all that, you can get lead disease." Carlton also bemoans the lack of fresh air in London, as compared with Barbados, Manchester or Cambridge. Louise says the same thing, adding that she was happiest in a small town in the Midlands.

Many of the informants have a rosy view of life somewhere else. Delores, Carlton and Donna all believe that Barbados is a much healthier place that Britain. Delores complains that in Britain, people are virtually housebound for most of the year, and that they cannot sit out to do their work and have a chat as she could in Barbados. She thinks, "the pressure, noise, aches and pains, too many pills and the weather, especially the cold weather" all contribute to her fading health in Britain. She goes on to say that her health is , "going down now in this country", and says that if she were in Barbados, she would deal with her ill-health with herbs, "but here, the slightest thing and you gotta go to the doctor. Everything is pills-pills-pills" (Delores). Her memories of Barbados are filled with healthiness - she says that no-one in her family was ever ill. Martha says the same, and Emily's and Millie's memories of Ghana are similarly free of ill-health. Nostalgic memories seem to help to alleviate some of the unpleasantnesses of life in Britain, today.

Donna and Carlton agree with their mother that living in Britain can damage a person's health: "In this country, as you get older, your health really suffers, but like old people in warmer countries like Barbados, you can't tell someone's age, but here, in England, you look older before your time. I think mostly it's to do with the cold weather: as you get older, you feel it, and things get harder for you. In warm countries it's just not like that - no rheumatic pain and stuff ... So many old people suffer here, from the cold weather. If they could just live in the warm sunshine, they would be all right - well, they wouldn't be cured, but they'd be better off" (Donna); "Now I see that my own parents might start to have rheumatism which is not really right for coloured people ... so that's definitely tellin' me that I will have it if I stay here too long. Nobody in Barbados suffers from rheumatism. They don't die out of pain, they die of old age, which is much more natural" (Carlton).

Jean, Ruby and Joe also think that the Caribbean is a healthier place in which to live. Joe feels that he is not so lively here, because he cannot exercise so easily here, and because of the lack of sunshine and fresh food. Jean figures that the sunshine, fresh food and the sea would make her much healthier if she went "home". Ruby says, "oh yes, the work make me sick, cold weather", and the fact that she cannot eat food when she wants to because the matron has stopped them from eating the kitchen left-overs.

Housing is not perceived to be a problem by many of the informants. Emily and Judy are the only ones who really want to live somewhere else: Emily because she cannot cope with eight flights of stairs, and Judy because her flat is, "situated funny", and the central heating does not work. Martha, Emily, Louise, Judy, Carlton, Earl, Leroy, Ruby and Delores all live in council flats, and although they are all beautifully kept inside, some of them are on old and overcrowded estates. Delores feels her first floor flat is like a bungalow in Barbados. Joe, Jean, Ivy, Danny and Paul live in mortgaged houses, and Donna in a mortgaged flat. Those who are buying their houses say that they prefer to own than to rent.

The council blocks are mainly pre- or immediately post-1945 blocks, most are recently modernised with central heating, but they are up to five stories high and none has lifts. Most of the informants agree that the sort of housing a person has can affect their health, and Delores, Leroy, and Carlton remember that they used to get a lot of colds when they lived in a damp flat. Dampness is singled out to be particularly injurious to health, and Delores and Earl feel that the central heating has to be just right, because places that are too warm are just as bad as those that are too cold. Temperature, as indicated above, is an important sign of ill-health.

There are other factors about living in Britain that are perceived to affect health. The reliance on pills rather than liquid medicines and herbal treatments is mentioned by some. Also involved are the conditions of work, the tinned and frozen food relied upon here, the lack of exercise, the lack of sunshine and freedom to go out lightly clothed. All of these are balanced against an idealised version of places once lived in or recently visited, such as the Caribbean, America or parts of Africa. None of the informants manages to suggest any benefits to health of living in Britain.

The Health Services

NHS Doctors and Drugs

All the informants are registered with an NHS general practitioner, chosen either because of the nearness of the surgery to their present or past homes (Delores, Ruby, Judy, Martha, Emily, Donna, Leroy and Carlton), or on the recommendation of a friend or relative (Ivy, Millie), or on the recommendation of another doctor (Joe, Jean, Danny, Paul). Ivy and Millie are quite prepared to travel long distances to see their doctor - Millie has to catch two buses. Earl also travels back to his original doctor. Both Earl and Millie have separate doctors for their children who go to the nearest surgery.

Some of the surgeries are single-handed (Delores, Leroy, Carlton, Ruby, Donna), and most operate on a "come and wait" basis. The surgery Judy attends, however, is a health centre, and she finds that she can choose between just turning up for emergencies (usually for her children), and making appointments (usually for herself). The surgery that Joe, Jean, Danny, Paul and Earl attend has three doctors and an appointments' system.

There are many complaints about the doctors and their surgeries. Leroy thinks the doctor should have more equipment (this is because of the failure of the doctor to diagnose his mother correctly - see below), and he feels the waiting system is unfair. Almost all the informants complain about the length of time they are obliged to wait. For some, the waiting puts them off going at all: "I don't like waitin' when I'm sick. I'd rather jus' go home, sleep it off" (Carlton); "I don't like havin' to go there when you're not feelin' well, and then havin' to wait" (Danny). As for improvements, no-one specifies any, but Ivy sums up their attitude when she says, "Improvements? What a chance when Maggie T'atcher's cuttin' down on the health service so you're not even sure of gettin' the right treatment these days."

Many mention the closure of local hospitals or casualty departments in their discussions about the health service. It is particularly worrying for some who now have to travel several miles by different bus routes to reach open A & E departments.

Most of the informants say initially that they are pleased with their GPs and are happy to stay with them, but in their stories about instances of ill-health and treatment, they are more critical. This public declaration of the value of doctors and, at the same time, holding of negative views about them has been found elsewhere (Cornwell, 1984). Straight-forward questions, such as, "Are you happy with your GP?" are usually met by publically-acceptable answers of, "yes", or, "of course." In-depth, informal interviewing techniqes, however, can expose people's deeper, private views (see Cornwell, 1984). Of these informants, only Ivy, Millie, Judy and Ruby are really happy with their GPs. Ivy says, for example, "I ask and he tells me ... I don't want to take something I don't know what it's for."

The criticisms of the doctors vary. The older women, particularly Ivy, Delores, Ruby and Martha say that they think doctors should examine them thoroughly. Ruby's doctor does these examinations and so she is happy, but the other women's doctors do not. Delores feels examinations are essential for, "inside problems or your periods." She refers particularly to the failure of her GP to diagnose her fibroids which eventually led to her having an emergency hysterectomy via a private doctor. She recalls that her GP, "never examine me, she jus' question me and say it could be the change of life." After several months of pain and discomfort, Delores eventually lost patience with the doctor's intransigence and went to her sister's private doctor.

Emily is reasonably happy with her doctor because he has agreed to visit her regularly. Louise is not happy with hers: "I don't like to go to surgery, and I don't go very often. When you go there, it is a waste of time. So many people, so many. For me to go there, it is very important. We have to sit down and wait for your turn - ages you have to wait." Donna is very critical of her previous doctor, the one who failed to diagnose her mother properly: "You go in and say this is wrong and then she'll start writing straight away. She never looks at you ... She don't explain. Like they say all these words and they don't tell you exactly what it means."

Like Donna, the men are very critical of doctors. Joe says, for example, "I hate doctors ... If I have a cold or a slight temperature, I would never tell the doctor." The younger men complain: "The thought of goin' to the doctor doesn't appeal to me unless I have to ... They've got more time for the elderly and infirm" (Paul); "I don't often see the doctors ... I haven't really got time ... It's just, 'What's the matter?' A swift exam., and tablets and away" (Danny); "I always wait until I have to go - really crawlin' in pain" (Leroy); "They don't seem to take an interest in what you've got. It's just, 'Oh! You've got this, I'll give you so many pills to take' ... If the doctor doesn't have proper contact with the patient, there's no point in going" (Earl).

The men are particularly annoyed and dissatisfied with the relationship they have with their doctors. Earl says, for example, that, "They could spend more time with the patient, break down the problem easier, diagnose it better ... You're in and out before you've had a chance to tell him what's wrong ... Doctors should be more versatile, visit people in their homes, see the conditions they're livin' in, what kind of stresses they're under." His friends, Leroy and Carlton agree:

"She's [the GP] controlling it [the consultation]. When I go in, I feel shy and I don't speak up and say what's wrong, what I think is wrong. She asks questions and I jus' answer them. Then she scribbles out a thing for you ... I come out of the doctors, I look at it, and, 'What am I sufferin' from?' ... You always know she's the doctor, and you're like, like a little kid" (Leroy); "I like to know what's wrong with me, what's goin' on and what I have to do. Not jus'. 'There's your prescription - take that!'" (Carlton).

Almost all of the informants were vague about when they last saw their general practitioner. Only Emily had seen hers within two weeks of the interview, when he had visited her about a throat infection and 'flu. Jean has never seen her present doctor, but all the others could remember going to the doctor and the reason for their visit, but they could not recall exactly when it was. Most had gone for minor complaints such as 'flu, stomach upsets, constipation and throat infections.

There is much evidence to suggest that going to the surgery is a last resort. Many of the informants have at their disposal a selection of home remedies that they trust to work (see remedies section). It is clear from what the men say, above, that they often delay going to see their doctor until they have to ,and this is also true of the women. Ivy says, "I delayed goin' to the doctor about me hypertension because I don't like tablets and I don't like botherin' the doctor. I'd rather use my 'bayrum'." Others say: "I couldn't be bothered. I didn't go ... I don't like visitin' doctors" (Jean); "You rub yourself down in the night and get a nice hot bath, and in the morning, it's OK, so you go to work, don't bother with the doctor" (Delores); "I don't go very often to the doctor ... you just get a common pain in your arm or knee, ankle, you try your own remedy - you just get something and you massage it in. If it get worse, you jus' <u>bear</u> it" (Martha).

Despite their professed abhorrance of drugs, only nine of the informants were not taking any drugs at the time of the life-story interview. Of the seven who admitted taking something, five of these are taking some long-term preparations for anaemia (Emily), asthma (Ruby), blood pressure (Ivy and Delores), hypertension (Ivy), depression or ulcer (Joe), and sugar diabetes (Ruby). Judy and Millie were taking panadols. The majority on long-term prescriptions, however, do not take their prescribed doses: Ivy is prescribed, "four each time, that is twelve a day, but now I jus' take one of each when I feel I need it. I decide"; Delores is prescribed three tablets per day, "and I don't always take 'em - only when I go to work"; Emily says, "I take iron, folic acid and ascorbic acid tablets. I been takin' one a day, but really I should take three a day, like I did when I came from hospital"; and Joe says, "sometimes I take 'em, and sometimes, I don't ... As long as I can get to work for Monday mornin', that's all right." Some of the informants also believe that NHS prescriptions are not very reliable. Ivy suggests, for example, that NHS drugs are, "just the dust of the main thing." She believes that the drugs her husband obtained from a private doctor were much better, more effective, and, presumably, the "main thing".

On the whole, then, the general practitioners are used, but usually after all else has been tried first. There are many complaints about the system, but few of the informants can see it being changed, although most would like to see it re-organised. More time, more doctors, examinations, and the chance to express their own views are the most important demands. Several would also like to see a recognition of, and sensitivity to, their own methods of health-care.

NHS Hospitals and the NHS

All of the informants have had some experience of hospital treatment, and they are divided almost equally over whether or not they were happy with the treatment they received. Delores, Jean, Earl, Joe, Paul, Louise and Emily are all pleased with their treatment. Delores, Emily and Louise had hysterectomies (Louise also had a mastectomy), and have very few complaints about hospital treatment: "Great! I'll always praise the doctors and nurses" (Delores). Jean received treatment for a broken foot, Earl for a torn ear, and Joe and Paul accompanied one of Joe's other sons to hospital after an accident with a fire extinguisher. None of these has any specific complaints.

Although being happy with their actual operations, Delores, Emily and Martha do complain about the time it took for their conditions to be diagnosed. Delores visited her GP for about a year, before she lost patience and consulted a private specialist. Emily recalls that she had felt tired for some months and had had a D&C [dilation and cutterage] in hospital, "and they didn't find anything wrong", but that only a few months later, she was diagnosed extremely anaemic and in need of a hysterectomy. She was too anaemic to have the operation for five or six months.

Martha says that she suffered more than three years of associated problems before her thyroid trouble was eventually cured. When asked whether or not she thought it should have been diagnosed earlier, she replies: "Not 'should've known', but I think in my case, it should've come to light earlier. It was eighteen months before they started proper treatment" (Martha).

Donna's personal experience of hospital treatment is limited to when she had her daughter, when she feels she was treated well, but otherwise, she says, "Talkin' about other people's experiences, I don't think it's all that good. You go along and you have to wait a long time. You could be bleeding, you still have to wait for someone to see you ... You wait such a long time for these other doctors and they haven't got time to talk to you or anything." Leroy's dissatisfaction arises from a lump on his wrist that bothers him when he works. He went into hospital to have it removed, but he had drunk a cup of tea beforehand and so they refused to operate. Since then, he has heard nothing. Carlton's complaint is similar: an injury he sustained in a car crash was being treated in hospital, and he says, "I had to go back every first of the month for injection ... I was gettin' fed up of goin' up to the hospital ... Didn't tell me what they was doin'." Consequently, he stopped the treatment, and cleared up the injury with a home remedy: coconut cream from Barbados.

Judy's complaints arise from her visit to hospital for a severe headache. On the whole, she is pleased with the hospital treatment for her sons, but had one unpleasant experience herself. She says that she eventually went to hospital after having a severe headache for just over a day, and that it had become, "unbearable." The doctor she saw told her to go home and to stop complaining. Millie recalls a similar incident in the same hospital. Millie went for period pains, only to be told that the hospital did not deal with period pains. She suspects that the doctor turned her away, "because he doesn't like blacks" (Millie). Later that day, Millie was rushed to hospital in a state of collapse and was detained for more than a week.

Millie's interview consists mainly of a story she wanted to tell about some treatment she received at a succession of north London hospitals. She is extrememly angry and upset, and her story does not make pleasant reading. It raises, however, many important issues. Millie believes quite clearly that negligence after the birth of her third child and later NHS procedures are directly to blame for her need to have a hysterectomy at the age of 33 years. It is worth bearing in mind that the child has sickle-cell anaemia, and although Millie is aware of the seriousness of the illness, she has not had explained to her the origin of the condition, nor that she must be a carrier of sickle-cell trait (see chapter three).

Her story is best told largely in her own words: "My trouble started when Ekow was born in hospital "A", and the doctors didn't come to see me ... not for four or five days, and I pass this big clot ... Den, after five days, a doctor came and apologised to me and says he's supposed to look after me, but they have emergencies ... After two more days, they check me up and tell me everything is all right. But since that day this boy was born, I am not the same."

"When I was in hospital, they ask me if I want family plannin'. I say, 'Yes.' When I went to the post-natal clinic, well they fitted me with this coil - they <u>supposed</u> to check me up, but they didn't check, jus' fix me coil. When she was doin' it, I didn't know what she was doin'. I thought she's examine me or somethin'. When she finish, she say, 'I have fix you a beautiful coil', and I say, '<u>WHAT!</u>' I shout, 'After six weeks? That ain't right.' ... She says, 'It's beautiful.' I say, 'It don't bother me whether it's beautiful or not, I come for a check up."

Millie confirms throughout that the coil was inserted without her knowledge, let alone her permission, and that the doctors were also completely ignorant of, and insensitive to, her cultural preferences and practices. She says, "Back 'ome, when you have a baby, you don't sleep with a man for may be three to six months, but here, after three or four weeks they go back to their husbands. We don't do that. I was waitin' until three or four months when I know I'm fit to sleep with a man."

She continues: "Since then, whenever I see my period, I get pain. I get pain. Never in my life did I have period pain ... So, I went to hospital "A". So they take it [the coil] out and fix me with another one. I say, 'I don't want another one', but they already fix it. Because I always use 'Miss', because I am not married, so they think they have a right to do what they did." She insists that no-one explained to her what they were doing: "Explain? <u>NO!</u> They fix me before they explain."

The month after this second coil was fitted, Millie again experienced terrible pain and was taken to hospital, given a D&C, and then fitted with another coil - again, she says, without her permission. Three months later, she attended hospital "B" with more severe pain, and they agreed to remove the coil, but, "They made me ready for the doctor and then they say that I have fibroids. I say, 'Fibroids? That was the coil then', for in my life I never had period problem except for the moment they fix me this coil."

Millie thought that hospital "B" had dealt with the fibroids, but two months later, she collapsed in pain and was taken to hospital "C", where, "they say I have got fibroids! I say, 'I can't, 'cause they have taken my fibroids out' ... but they insist." She was put on the waiting list, but again she collapsed and spent seven days in hospital "C", where they, "make me ready to have a hysterectomy. I say, 'What?' They say, 'Yes,or you won't get better.' I couldn't believe it - I was 33, but I says OK, 'cause I know what I'm sufferin'" (Millie).

Millie is the most critical of NHS hospitals, and she is most critical of all of hospital "A", a north London hospital with a world-wide reputation. She says, "It's useless. Damn useless. They are doin' big, big research; dey haven't got time for me, for headaches. If you go in with your small, small disease, you will die there."

Several of the informants think that the NHS is a waste of money, and they complain that far from being free, it costs them quite a lot of money through their national insurance payments. Paul, Danny, Donna and Carlton hold this view. Delores has mixed opinions, disliking the way she has to pay for it, but not wanting it to be disbanded altogether.

Joe feels that the NHS should change its outlook, "by studyin' tropical roots and bushes to find new remedies and cures." Since the health-workers dispute was on at the time of the majority of the interviews, most informants mention the hardworking staff, and how, "they are grossly underpaid" (Earl). The informants' opinions on the NHS and its hospitals depends largely upon their experience of it. The majority have been well treated and have favourable or neutral opinions about it, and a few have had unpleasant experiences and hold negative views about it.

Private Medicine

The lack of faith in the NHS exhibited by the informants is linked with their views on private treatment. Only one says clearly that he would not go to a private doctor if he had "free choice" (Leroy), and two others say that they can see no reason to go while there is still an NHS (Emily and Louise). The others all suggest that they would either prefer an entirely private health system, like there is in the USA, or just that they like to see private doctors, if the NHS, "Couldn't give me my satisfaction" (Jean).

Of those who would prefer to see a private doctor, only four have actually seen one. Martha was recommended a private doctor, and she went to see him once about the menopause, but she says, "The doctors are the same - no better, no worse. Just the same ... I wouldn't go again." Delores, Ivy and Ruby are the others to have consulted private doctors, to, "get a run down" (Delores); "for the same old check up jus' to see if my system is workin' OK" (Ivy). Ruby says, "sometimes I jus' cyan't go to the National doctor", and her preference for a private doctor is reinforced by her view that Delores could have died if she had not seen a private doctor.

These women do not go to the same private doctor on a regular basis, but choose the doctor according to the look of the premises. The private surgeries are thought to be, "more like a house ... Up to date lookin'" (Ivy). The doctors, they say, give them more time, are willing to give them full "run-down" examinations, and to explain what is wrong and what prescriptions they needs. Ivy suggests, "You're payin' out, and you expect to get your money's worth." They also believe that the private drugs are better: "They give you somethin' different of what the national doctor would give, and sometimes they give you more. You haffi keep goin' back to the national doctor, but sometimes the private doctor will give you an injection and dat cure it" (Ruby); "The drugs are much stronger than the NHS, because you pay more money", and NHS prescriptions, "are just the dust of the main thing" (Ivy).

Those who have not actually visited a private doctor say that they are willing to, because, "money talks" (Paul); the private doctors, "Devote more time to you because you are payin' them to offer you a service" (Earl); "On the NHS you get treated anyhow because you're not payin'" (Judy). Donna feels that private doctors will treat a person properly, "because you're payin' them to do a complete run down on you." Four of the informants would prefer to see a private doctor, but are constrained by lack of money: Judy, Jean, Earl and Danny, who says that private medicine, "is for a very different class of person." On the whole, though, the verbal preference for private treatment is only matched in practice by four of the older women who have had experience of health care in the West Indies, where treatment has to be paid for. Most are reluctant to pay out for health care when they already pay national insurance, and few would acually like to see the NHS disbanded in favour of a private scheme because as Donna says, since not everyone can afford to pay, the NHS, "might be good for some people."

CONCLUSION

These, then, are the perceptions and experiences of health, ill-health and the health services of the informants of Afro-Caribbean descent. Of particular importance to their health are work, religion, racism, chance, fate, food, germs, worries, remedies, exercise, depression and the quality of the treatment they receive. Some of these are perceived to act against good health, notably racism, germs and worries. Others cause ill-health, but are also perceived to have beneficial effects, such as work; and others have perceived beneficial effects on health, such as remedies, religion and exercise.

The health of the informants is largely determined by things outside their control, such as the jobs they have, the places they live, the racial discrimination they suffer, the germs they catch, and the course that episodes of ill-health take. Some resign themselves to having very little, if any, control or choice over their lives and health, relying instead on religious beliefs, or just accepting "the way things are." Others feel that they can exercise some control and choice by keeping fit to ward off ill-health, by eating the right foods and taking the "proper" precautions. Once ill-health has set in, there is a general acceptance of its effects, but many of the informants employ remedies to ease symptoms or cure conditions, or turn to religion for its psychological and psychosomatic effects.

In sum, then, the health of the informants, like their lives, is largely determined by broad social, economic and political forces in Britain, in combination with the action of disease-carrying agents such as germs. The informants' defence against these forces is chiefly cultural: they can use traditional foods to build up the strength of the body, employ remedies for specific conditions, practise a chosen religion which gives them a sense of peacefulness and strength, or do sports to keep the body in good condition so that it can ward off some germs. There is, thus, some individual power within the overarching societal constraints acting on them.

The next chapter is concerned with the perceptions and experiences of health, ill-health and the health services of the informants of Asian descent. Further categorisation of the material in this chapter and chapter six will be left until chapter seven, in which the similarities and differences between the two groups will be considered, and the links between the introductory chapters (one to four) and the empirical work (five and six) will be made more explicit.

6 The perceptions and experiences of the Asian informants

The Informants

As with the Afro-Caribbean informants in chapter five, the informants of Asian descent were obtained according to the key informant and snowball sampling strategies. The first, and key, informant (Naseem) was contacted through a social worker who was known to be interested in health and who worked in an area with a relatively large Asian population. The social worker initially invited me to observe a meeting of Asian women about issues of health and the NHS in a local club. I was introduced to the women, but as the meeting was conducted in Hindi and I could speak no Asian languages, I could not arrange to interview anybody.

The social worker arranged for me to visit Naseem a few days later as she was known to speak several languages (including English) and was interested in my project. I first visited Naseem in January, 1983. The visit was successful, and Naseem offerred to act as an interpreter for me and to approach her friends/acquaintances to become informants. Naseem thus became the key informant for the Asian group, and formed the origin of the little snowball sampling that did occur. Naseem subsequently arranged all the interviews. I organised transport by taxi where necessary and ensured that Naseem would be paid a fair rate for her work as an interpreter.

Naseem was herself interviewed in English in January, 1983. Three days later, we visited her next-door neighbour, Taresh. In February, six women were interviewed: Syeda, Rani, Tasneem, Sufiya, Farah, Farida and Dalee. The remaining five women were seen in March: Geeta, Shobha, Baji, Rajinda and Reena. I asked to interview some men, but all of the women said that their husbands were too busy or available only late in the evening. Only Rani's husband was present during the interview with his wife, and this was because only one room was then habitable owing to alterations to the house. On the whole, the women enjoyed being the centre of attention and seemed not to want to involve their husbands.

All of the women interviewed were born outside Britain: Tasneem, Farida, Dalee, Geeta, Baji, Rajinda and Reena in India; Naseem, Taresh, Syeda, Rani, Sufiya and Farah in Pakistan; and Shobha in Kenya. Their ages range from eighteen to "in the region of sixty to seventy" - the oldest woman being unsure of her age. Most of the women are married and have children. Only Farida, who is eighteen, is not married, and only Rani of the married women has no children of her own.

After her interview, Naseem gave advice as to which points and questions were suitable and which needed simplification, omission or addition. The questions generally used are similar to those for the women of Afro-Caribbean descent (see Appendix I), although the bracketed questions were added to be asked only of the women of Asian descent. These concern issues of language.

The first interview with Naseem acting as an interpreter was with Taresh, her next-door neighbour. At first, I asked Naseem to interpret each sentence as it was spoken, but it became clear that this broke up the flow of what the informant wanted to say, and Naseem found it difficult to interrupt, then interpret, listen for a short while and then interrupt again. Some of this interview was, therefore, lost while an adequate technique was developed. In the end, it seemed best that Naseem should listen to the story the informant was telling, and then interpret it for my benefit. In this way, Naseem was able to make sense of the story, to check it with the informant, and then I was able to follow up stories as I had done with the informants of Afro-Caribbean descent. The whole of the interview, including Naseem's interpretations, was tape-recorded, and the passages in English were fully transcribed.

The relationships of the informants to Naseem and each other are set out in Fig 6(i). Some biographical details of the women are set out in Tables 6(i) and 6(ii).

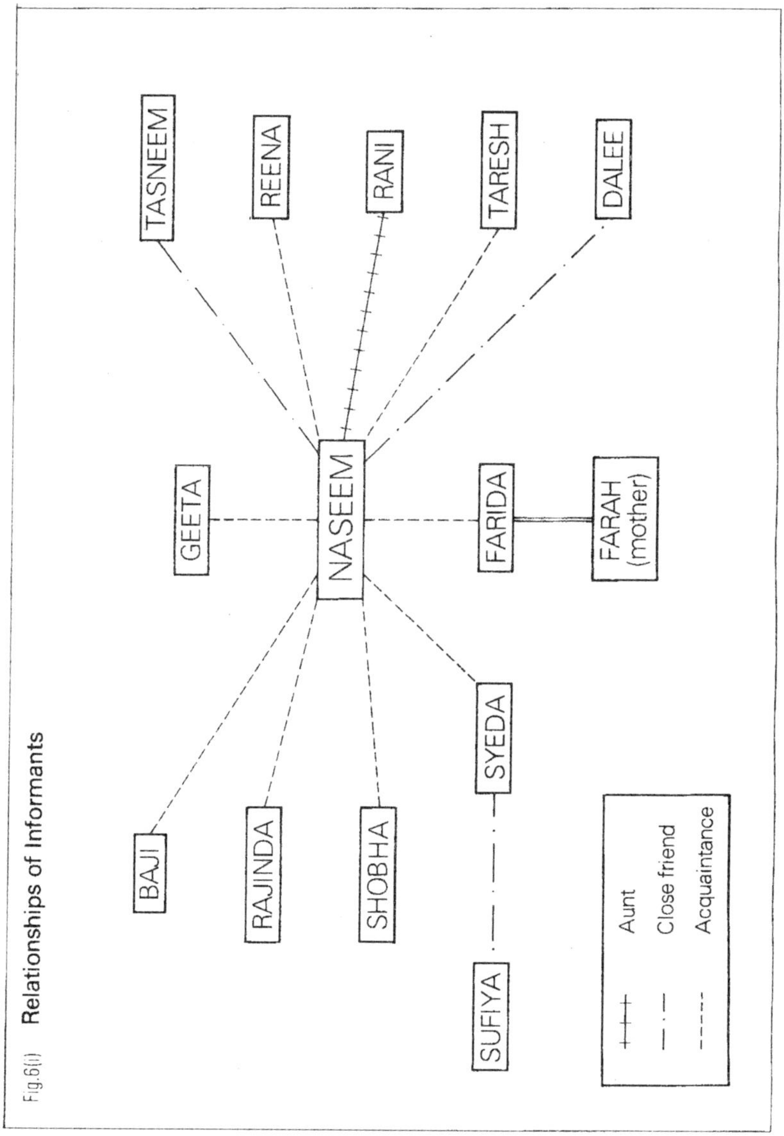

Fig.6(i) Relationships of Informants

Table 6(i) Some Biographical Details of the Informants

NAME	PLACE OF BIRTH	AGE	LANGUAGE**	MARITAL STATUS	NUMBER OF CHILDREN
Tasneem	India	34	Urdu/English	M	4
Farida	India	18	Urdu	S	0
Dalee	India	38	Urdu/English	M	2
Geeta	India	60-70*	Gujerati	M	4
Baji	India	50	Punjabi	M	7
Rajinda	India	28	Punjabi	W	1 (deceased)
Reena	India	55*	Punjabi	M	8
Naseem	Pakistan	43	English	M	2
Taresh	Pakistan	27	Urdu	M	3
Syeda	Pakistan	28	Urdu	M	4***
Rani	Pakistan	57	Urdu	M	0****
Sufiya	Pakistan	27	Urdu/English	M	2
Farah	Pakistan	42	Urdu	M	4
Shobha	Kenya	34	English/Urdu	M	3

Notes

See notes for Table 5(i)

* These informants were unsure of their age.

** The language(s) mentioned are the ones used in the interviews. Where there are two, the first indicated was the most often used during the interviews.

*** Rani has two adopted children.

**** Due to an error on my part, I omitted to ask any questions of Syeda about her pregnancies. Naseem had told me that one of the women had adopted her children because she could not have any of her own, and that no-one, including Naseem was supposed to know about this. Naseem asked, consequently, that I should not ask about her pregnancy history, and I thought (mistakenly) that Syeda was the woman to whom Naseem was referring. Unfortunately, it was Rani.

Table 6(ii) Some More Biographical Details of Informants

NAME	JOB	PARTNER'S JOB	HOUSE TYPE	LENGTH FIRST INTERVIEW	SECOND INTERVIEW
Tasneem		Factory owner	MH	1hr30m	yes
Farida			MH	- 15m	no
Dalee		Accountant	MH	1hr -	no
Geeta	Machine work	Retired carpenter	MH	- 45m	no
Baji		Own building business	MH	1hr -	no
Rajinda		Bus conductor	MH	2hr -	no
Reena		Builder	MH	1hr -	no
Naseem		Civil servant	MH	1hr15m	yes
Taresh	Machine work	Car assembler	MH	1hr -	no
Syeda		Factory inspector	MH	1hr -	no
Rani		Retired civil servant	MH	1hr -	yes
Sufiya		Own business	MH	1hr -	no
Farah		Civil servant	MH	- 30m	no
Shobha	Machine work	Foreman builder	MH	- 45m	yes

Notes

See notes for Table 5(ii)

During the interviews I tried to be aware of the effects I might be having on the responses of the informants. Naseem had told me that many of the women were very religious and did not approve of clothes which exposed the limbs, and so to ensure that I did not to embarrass the women, particularly Naseem, I always wore trousers and clothes of modest designs and colours. When the women asked why I was doing the research project, I always told them that I was a student who was interested in what they thought about health, illness and the health services. Some asked why I was speaking to them, and I explained that although research had been done on the health of Asian people, very little had actually focused on their thoughts and opinions.

Usually on these visits, Naseem and I were offered food and drink, and we always accepted. Sometimes this occurred during the interviews, sometimes after, and when it was the latter, I was usually asked about my background. As with the women of Afro-Caribbean descent, the Asian women were particularly interested in what it was like to be Jewish, as well as the death of my father at an early age. Several were also concerned about what they considered to be my low weight, and were interested to know that I do not eat meat. Several were also interested in my education history and what sort of degree I was doing; and some went on to liken me to a young relative of theirs also doing a degree of some sort.

Quite often during the interviews, the women asked my opinions about the questions I was asking them, some of them seeing me at first as "an expert". Whenever this happened, I emphasised my student status and my youth, and gave the best answers I could. I always tried to give my comments after they had given theirs, so as to minimise the effects of what I had said.

The use of an interpreter was an important factor in most of the discussions. This was unavoidable in many cases because I did not want to leave out those women who did not speak English, and even some of those who were able to answer some questions in English preferred to use an Asian language to tell stories or convey complex thoughts. As Naseem was known to all the women, either through the local club or by living nearby, as an educated woman and one who would help most of them fill in forms, write letters and even teach some of them English, she was able to put the other women at ease. As a friend and/or relative of some of the women, she could also probe some sensitive issues, although in some cases she was unwilling to ask questions if she knew they might offend the woman involved. I attended some Urdu classes, and could sometimes understand the gist of what was being said so that in some cases I knew what to expect of Naseem's interpretations. Since several of the women could speak English, but interrupted rarely, and since Rani's husband was present but altered very few of Naseem's interpretations, I feel confident that Naseem interpreted effectively.

The tape-recorder was sometimes intrusive at the beginning of interviews, and all the women except Geeta asked why I was using it. Some were worried that I might take down their family details and inform the police, but once Naseem and I explained that the tape-recorder was only an aid to me, that I did not want to know their names, and that I would be the only person to listen to the tapes, nobody objected. After initial reservations, no-one was concerned about the use of the tape-recorder.

All the informants were asked about their life-stories. Four were, at a later date, involved in the more focused talk. Naseem, being the key informant was interviewed first in English. Again I relied on Naseem to tell of any unsuitable questions. The only question that she thought was impossible was, "Is there any difference between an illness and a disease?" In Urdu, the word "beemaar" means illness, disease, trouble and problem with little differentiation. This question was, therefore, dropped.

As with the informants of Afro-Caribbean descent, those of Asian descent proved difficult to revisit. After Naseem was seen, the weather became bad, and so they were postponed. When we attempted to re-start the interviews in December, 1983 the women were all too busy with religious festivals such as Mohammed's birthday, and no-one could spare the time. Eventually, Naseem persuaded Rani to be seen again, and this time her home was finished and very comfortable. Rani's husband was again present, but he interrupted very little, and when he began to tell a story of his own, Rani swiftly silenced him.

The focused discussions with Rani and Tasneem were conducted entirely in Urdu because the points were difficult for them to express in English. Naseem spoke only English, and Shobha used both English and Urdu. Shobha's discussion was constrained by her need to return to her sewing machine work, and she was able only to give us twenty-five minutes of her time.

The interviews with Tasneem and Rani were all somewhat overshadowed by the shock of another illness to their (and Naseem's) close friend, Dalee. She had been planning to go to Pakistan for a holiday, but had suffered another stroke on the evening before she was due to leave because, according to Naseem and Tasneem, she had stopped taking her prescribed steroids. The stroke has left Dalee blind, and there is only a fifty-fifty chance that she will regain her sight. Their friend's sudden stroke has shocked the women and is reflected paticularly in their answers to questions such as, "Are there any illnesses you are afraid of getting?" Their answers to these questions must be seen, therefore, in the context of their shocked reaction to Dalee's stroke.

As with the previous chapter, the material from the focussed questions and the life-story interviews has been combined. The material has been broken into the same categories and sections as chapter five, the broad sections being concerned with: the informants' medical histories; the perceptions of health and ill-health; the causes of ill-health; the perceived severity of conditions; the general effects of "culture" on lifestyle and health; the effects of living in Britain; and the informants' experiences of the health services in Britain. These are reported below.

Health and Illness in Their Lifetimes : An Introduction

Table 6(iii)
Outline of Major Episodes of Ill-Health in Selected Informants' Lives

NAME	SURGERY	SERIOUS ILL-HEALTH	MINOR ILL-HEALTH
Naseem		Coeliac disease	Period problems
		Slipped disc	Leg pains
Tasneem		Typhoid (child)	Diarrhoea
		TB	
Rajinda		[Husband shot dead]	Headaches
		[Daughter died in mysterious way]	Skin problems
			Period problems
Rani	Gall-bladder	Typhoid (child)	Strained back
Dalee		Rheumatoid arthritis	Broken arm
		High blood pressure	
		Paralysis. Strokes	
		"SLE"	
		Temporary blindness	
Sufiya		Smallpox (child)	Headaches
			Skin problems
Taresh			Headaches
			Period problems
Reena		Cataracts	Headaches
Baji	Hysterectomy		Period problems
			Leg pains
Shobha		Anaemia	

All of the informants were asked about their health and the ill-health that they had suffered during their childhoods and up to the present. Table 6(iii) sets out the major episodes of ill-health in some of the informants' lives. Most of the women said that they were healthy children, but when asked about what illnesses or diseases they had actually had, several mention quite serious conditions. It is remarkable that these serious illnesses are accepted as part of life: "Sometimes I had sore eyes or fever or a headache ... I used to get malaria or fever"

(Sufiya); "As I grew up I was healthy ... I had typhoid when I was ten years old" (Baji); "When I was nine, I had typhoid - that's all" (Rajinda); "When I was five or six, I had serious kind of boil on my back" (Syeda). Sufiya also had smallpox as a child, and Tasneem and Rani both had typhoid. Geeta, Farida and Reena all claim to have been very healthy during their childhoods, having no illnesses. The others all mention "fever" as a common illness, caused by a, "change of season" (Taresh, Rani); or a, "change of weather" (Sufiya, Farah, Dalee); or, "mosquito" (Farah, Rani); or, "too much heat" (Reena, Rajinda).

Quite often a doctor or hakim (a practitioner of traditional medicine) was seen for the various episodes of ill-health suffered. Naseem's parents, for example, tried western doctors, homeopaths and hakims to discover the cause of Naseem's stomach troubles, but none of them could do anything but temporarily relieve the symptoms of bloating and nausea. The only other woman to admit using a hakim is Taresh, who says they were seen for, "minor illnesses, like temperature or 'flu." Hakims tend to be the practitioners for the poor because they sell cheap medicines, whereas the rich and those associated with the government and the military use western-style doctors and hospitals. Several of the group interviewed originally came from wealthy or government-associated families, and so few used hakims. None had seen a hakim in Britain, and several added that they did not think they practised over here, except for the occasional visit of a famous hakim from Pakistan.

Only Rani and Syeda were rich enough to go to hospital when they were children. Syeda had a boil removed from her back, and Rani went in when she was seriously ill with typhoid. Sometimes, they were visited by doctors: Sufiya for smallpox injections, and Baji for typhoid treatment. Most of the women say that ill-health was just coped with within the family: "We never used to go to the doctor or hakim when we were children ... We didn't ever <u>need</u> any medicine at all" (Reena), echoed by Geeta and Rajinda.

The informants do not remember many people being ill when they were children. Only four of the women say that they can remember specific instances of ill-health: Rani recalls that her mother died of heart failure; Dalee says that her father's family had sugar diabetes; and Syeda's mother and Tasneem's brother both had tuberculosis. The past in another country seems a long way off to the informants, and it may be that they are reluctant to look back because memories of their families and places they have not seen for so long upset them.

As with the Afro-Caribbean informants, the teenage years are not really distinct, and merge with the much more important events of marriage and pregnancy. This period is remembered by all the women as being a healthy one, especially since only the healthy women are allowed to marry. Naseem still had her "tummy troubles", but as they did not affect her too much, she was able to marry. Tasneem and Rani had typhoid around the ages of fifteen or sixteen, Tasneem particularly seriously: "I had a very high temperature for about three weeks and people said I was not going to live" (Tasneem), but in the end both recovered and were married.

Only two of the informants have no children of their own: Farida, who is unmarried, and Rani. Having children is seen as essential by the women, and sons are particularly highly valued. As Naseem had two sons, she was able to decide not to have any more children after the difficult birth of her sons. Syeda, however, who has four daughters, is still trying to have a son. She is especially upset at the time of the interview because she had recently had a miscarriage. Sufiya's worries about her son's health (he has thalassaemia and a hole in the heart) are compounded by the fact that he is her only son.

Seven of the women had all their pregnancies in Britain (Naseem, Taresh, Tasneem, Sufiya, Dalee, Shobha and Rajinda), and all but Taresh had all their deliveries in London hospitals - Taresh had one child while on a visit to Pakistan. None has any complaints about having to have children in hospital, but there are some specific comments on their treatment which are dealt with in the section on NHS hospitals. Three women had all their pregnancies and deliveries in India (Farah, Baji and Reena), and one did so in Kenya (Geeta). Only Reena and Geeta, the two oldest women, had all their deliveries at home with a midwife, and Baji had her last twins at home when she could not reach the hospital. Otherwise, all the deliveries were in hospital. Tasneem, Syeda and Dalee report that they have had miscarriages, and Geeta and Reena had children who died soon after birth.

Most of the women say that their pregnancies were normal and went well. Most saw a doctor regularly, but only Dalee and Tasneem went to ante-natal classes in Britain. None really did anything specific to keep themselves healthy during pregnancy, apart from trying to eat good food, such as fresh fruit and vegetables, milk and butter. Only Farah reports taking a tonic: "I used to have milk with almond powders, and in the morning I used to have apple jam. This was a tonic for the pregnancy. The mother-in-law told me it was a good thing."

A time that is not remembered with pleasure by many of the informants is the period of migration and settlement in Britain. For a few, it was not too bad because their husbands had been settled for some time and had everything arranged for them (Rani, Geeta). Most of the women arrived to marry, or came with their parents, and almost all speak of the pain of leaving their families and friends behind. Much of the informants' depression originates from the time of immigration, and is exacerbated by the infrequency of visits abroad and the difficulties of communication. Farah and Farida are particuarly affected, having arrived in Britain only six weeks before they were interviewed. As the leaving date was fixed, and as the whole family came over, Farida had to leave university in the middle of her final year. She has little hope of taking up a course in Britain for some time because although she can write English, she cannot speak it.

The time of arrival is spoken of as one of terrible loneliness and a feeling of great loss. For some of the women it was also the time when they were newly married and so they found new domestic duties to become accustomed to as well as a new and strange place. Sufiya recalls, "I had to finish my schooling here and so it was not very pleasant in the beginning. I felt very lonely and ... I couldn't mix with the other girls because of the language, and everything is different to Pakistan." It was also a difficult time for Naseem: "It was a very, very painful experience for me to leave them [doting parents] and come to a completely strange country where I didn't have anybody, no relatives except my husband ... I just cried night and day and asked my husband to please send me back."

The initial shock of arrival has been tempered by time for most of the informants, but many still miss their relatives who are still abroad. Reena speaks particuarly of her daughter's husband who is being prevented from coming to Britain. When Reena's family were forced out of Kenya, all except her son-in-law had British passports, and so were obliged to come to Britain. The son-in-law had to go to India, an he has not managed to get into Britain in ten years. Reena is bitter: "We were forced out of Kenya, so we had to come here, but if we had Indian nationality, we would have gone to India rather than here."

This, then, is the background to their arrival in Britain. Most of the informants have been in Britain fewer than fifteen years. The majority of the interview time was, however, focused on the needs and concerns of the present or recent past. Although the material has been broken into sections, it is important to bear in mind that many of the issues raised are complex and interlinked.

Perceptions of Health and Illness

Definitions of health

Health is seen to be a state of perfection by most of the informants and is defined by the absence of ill-health. All the informants agree that good health is important to them, mainly so that they are able to look after their children and carry on with the housework. For a few, it is of more general importance: "You are only happy when you are healthy. If you are ill, nothing looks good to you" (Sufiya); "There is no life without health" (Farida); "Nobody likes to be ill" (Reena). For most of the women, and throughout the interviews, the importance of health is linked to the present-day concerns of the health of children and other relatives, and the need for strength to work or do housework.

None of the women believes that there can be anyone in the world who is perfectly healthy. Even Farida, who has not had any serious illnesses, has had some minor episodes of ill-health and has not, therefore, had perfect health. Perfect health is seen as an unattainable state where, "A person is completely healthy - no illness, no depression, and nothing wrong with the body" (Naseem); "When you are able to do everything as you can. Whatever you want to do and you have no illness, no pains, nothing" (Rani); "When you are perfectly relaxed and happy in your house" (Shobha).

Perfect health does not seem to exist for anyone because, "most of the time there is something that is making a person ill, psychologically" (Naseem); and as Rani adds, "whenever you have little bit of illness, you cannot say that you are healthy or that you are perfect." Naseem thinks that there are "some people who are quite healthy and quite happy in this world", but all the women agree with Rani when she says: "There is nobody who is perfectly healthy. For everybody there is something wrong somewhere, but if you have less worries, less tension, then may be you are better off. When you are young, you are much better, but as the age, with the time, you get certain illnesses and pains and aches. There is nobody in the world who could be called perfectly healthy" (Rani).

For several of the informants, the environment and social organisation of Britain is less conducive to perfect health than other places. In fact, even good health is seen to be almost unattainable in Britain because of the depression and worries caused by having relatives far away. Naseem also complains that health is at risk, "for we don't get any help in the home" - no servants, so all the domestic duties fall on the women. Tasneem has been influenced by some propaganda against Asian food, for she has heard that Asian women are particularly at risk of ill-health because they do not eat the right sort of food or cook it in the right ways. She adds that the lack of health is especially so "with the Asian ladies ... For a few years, some of them are all right, but after that, they get one or the other ailment." This theme is developed in later sections.

The health of the informants at the time of the life-story interview varies. For some, they are, "All right" or, "Not too bad, really" (Naseem, Taresh, Shobha, Syeda and Rani). Others have almost perfect health: "I can't remember when I was last ill" (Farah); "I've never been ill" (Farida); "Since I came to this country, I've never been ill" (Geeta). Thus "health" is chiefly seen as a residual condition, a state of not being ill.

Definitions of Ill-Health

Although there are several words in English to denote the presence of ill-health, this is not the case in the Asian languages spoken by the informants. The word, "beemaar", covers the concepts of illness, sickness, disease and problem, so the issue of the difference between an illness and a disease does not arise. Only Naseem, who speaks fluent English is able to distinguish between these two concepts, and she is not sure: "If you are mentally ill, that is called "illness". If you are physically ill, that is also "illness", but disease is caused by germs, I am sure, and that can be only physical."

The informants broadly agree over what an "illness" is: "The illness is when the person doesn't feel himself well enough to do all the things which the person has to do. Where he can't cope with everything - the housework or the job" (Naseem); "If you have got headache, you won't be able to do all your work as you possibly can; or if you have got pain in the body, you will not be able to perform your duties as you were usually doing. So, whenever that you have any sort of ailment, that would be called illness" (Rani); and "even if you have a little headache, you don't feel as normal as you should do. You think you are going to be ill" (Tasneem).

The last time the informants felt unwell was often not long before the interview. The most commonly mentioned illness was a headache, with four of the women saying that they suffer from them regularly. Two of these feel that their headaches may have some physical cause: "I feel sick ... The pain is just like somebody is beating you with a hammer inside the head" (Taresh), and she wonders if the cause may be related to her difficulties with a contraceptive coil; and Reena, who says, "I have severe kind of headaches. I have a cataract in the eyes as well and that might cause it. It's like a burning sensation in my head." Rajinda and Sufiya relate their headaches to psychological factors: Rajinda is depressed about her husband's death in an accident and her daughter's death: "I have no physical trouble, but whenever I think of that accident or my daughter in the night, the next morning I cannot get up, I get such a severe headache"; and Sufiya thinks her headaches are the result of her worries about her son's ill-health and her perennial tiredness.

Other complaints mentioned are period difficulties (Baji, Taresh and Naseem); leg pains (Naseem and Baji); circulation trouble (Taresh and Naseem); and skin disorders (Rajinda and Sufiya). The first signs that a person is ill are seen to be headaches, pain in the body and tiredness. Naseem says, "You feel tired, don't feel like doing any work. Sometimes you feel like you're getting a temperature. You will feel shivery or cold. If you have some sort of infection in the throat, you can feel it ... Or the pain in the chest. These kind of things tell you that you are not very well - are ill"; and Rani says, "If you feel headache or pain in the eyes or the body, or you feel tired, it means that you are feeling ill - that you are not as healthy as you were before."

Such are the definitions of health and ill-health among this group. The definition of a feeling as an illness, however, depends on the severity of the condition, its visibility, the social obligations of the time, and the person's experiences and heritage. Although the definitions elucidated above do hold on many occasions, their context is crucial in determining whether a condition is ignored, action is postponed, or action is taken and the condition eased.

The Causes of Ill-Health

The origins of episodes of ill-health are not things that the informants are particularly concerned with. Ill-health is usually accepted to "just happen", and the most important thing is seen to be to overcome it and to get on with life. The informants speculate on the causes of some conditions, however, and these often arise from cultural beliefs and perceptions (see also culture section).

Fate

Overall, there is a general acceptance of health and ill-health as part of life, with ill-health in particular being something to be expected and something that is almost impossible to prevent. Fatalism runs through many of the interviews, in connection with health and illness, and life itself. All the informants of Asian descent are religious to some degree, and the power of God's will is related to fate in determining what will happen to people and why. The acceptance of the way things are enables the informants to cope with ill-health and personal difficulties, and to get on with life.

Naseem sums up her feelings: "You can get ill, any time of your life. You can never expect that you will always be healthy. A mis-hap can happen, any time. You can get ill, you can get some disability by accident, because these things are in God's hands and everybody should expect that they will get ill, any time." This view is echoed by Shobha, and Rani continues, "One should expect that one can get sick any time because in the world, there is no-one who is perfectly healthy. When people are just walking on the streets or doing their job, they can just die, instantly." She goes on to describe, incredulously, the death of her previous GP in his surgery while he was attending his patients, and concludes, "so, you can expect anything, illness or death in this world, any time."

For some, an individual is thought to be able to prevent the onset of ill-health, but such precautions do not always work: "Only thing you can do is take care of yourself - if there is anything that makes you ill, avoid doing that ... We can just take care, but it depends on God. You can still get ill, any time" (Rani). Naseem agrees wholeheartedly: "There are some ways where you can help yourself to keep yourself fit and healthy, by eating proper food, having good sleep and good rest, but there are certain times when a person can't help for the health at all .. So, there are ways where you can keep yourself healthy, but there is no guarantee, you can still get ill sometimes."

The attitude of acceptance, fatalism and especially faith is summed up in many of the women's thoughts on their futures: "It is in the hands of God. Anything can happen to a person, anytime" (Taresh); "It is in God's hands ... I hope that until I die, I should be healthy, so I am no burden on anybody" (Geeta); "It is not in our hands - only God knows" (Reena). Religious beliefs thus crucially inderpin many of these informants' perceptions (see also, culture section).

Fault

The idea of personal responsibility for ill-health runs counter to the idea of fate and God's will controlling everything, but several of the women find that they can assign blame to some conditions. Rani is an exceptionally religious woman, and she cannot accept that people can cause their own illnesses: "Everybody wants to be healthy ... I don't think that anybody would think that it is somebody's fault that they are ill. It can't be. It can just happen."

Most of the other women, however, do acknowledge that illness can be brought on by individual action. Dalee, for example, speaks at length about her serious illness which has led to three strokes, and she firmly lays the blame for the first stroke on advice given to her by a homeopathic doctor which caused her to give up taking steroid drugs (see private medicine section). Similarly, Naseem accepts that her slipped disc was exacerbated and made into a permanent condition because, "The doctor told me to have two weeks' complete rest, but I couldn't because I had some guests from Pakistan and I also have my children. I had no help at all, so I had to get up, do the housework."

Tasneem feels that the influence of fate and fault is balanced: "Sometimes the illness is natural and sometimes it is the fault of your own ... Usually, it is natural, the illness. Most of the time it's not a person's fault." She believes that the incorrect sort of food or unnecessary worrying can bring on ill-health. Naseem has coeliac disease (an allergy to gluten), and so she knows that she will be ill if she eats any food containing gluten. Thus she can see that people can be responsible for their ill-health, sometimes: "I don't think that anybody would like to make himself or herself ill. It is not anybody's <u>fault</u>, it happens. Whatever has to happen, happens, you know. May be sometimes, if you are allergic to something and the doctors have stopped you from eating certain food and you still eat it, well then, that can be your fault, can't it? You will make yourself ill" (Naseem). Like the others, she feels that people should take expert advice and "proper" precautions to avoid becoming ill.

Worries

Throughout their interviews, some of the informants make a distinction between physical and mental health. Naseem, for example, believes that disease can only refer to physical ill-health, whereas "illness" can refer to physical or mental conditions. She continues, "The illness, if it is caused by some mental reason, then sometimes they can't find it out" (Naseem). Tasneem, her friend, concurs, "If you are physically healthy, sometimes you are mentally ill. People who are worried, they have got mental problems ... so they are ill in a way."

There is a close connection between the influence of worries and depression on health, and both are seen to be able to cause and exacerbate ill-health. Worries are seen more often as a cause of ill-health, usually mental ill-health, but with some physical manifestations. Reena, for example, says, "It is mostly worries that make a person ill ... If I worry about something or think about something, sometimes I feel very panicky, I start sweating and shaking." She is worried particularly about her daughter's husband who is unable to get into Britain owing to nationality difficulties, and it causes her to have, "pains in my knees and legs ... I am worried about my headaches and cataract ... If I sleep, I feel better, but I can't even sleep now because of this headache" (Reena). She misses the open fields of India and now has the added worry of a forthcoming cataract operation which terrifies her.

Rajinda is another of the women who reports a physical manifestation of worries. After the death of her husband, she says her in-laws have caused her trouble by telephoning her and, she claims, by setting fire to her car. They blame her for her husband's death, and she worries in case they should arrive and frighten her: "If anybody comes suddenly, I just start shaking ... I cannot get up from the chair, I can't move or do anything. My head feels funny. It's the pressure, the worry for me. I get headaches and pains and aches in the body" (Rajinda). This is some evidence, then, for the supposed somatisation of complaints by some people of Asian descent mentioned in chapter three.

Shobha, who has had some domestic difficulties in trying to prevent her husband's parents from living in their house, says, "Worries are the worst cause for the illness ... Any domestic problem, outside pressure from in-laws, husband or home, any kind of pressure can cause you illness." For her, then, her own experience is crucial. Tasneem agrees with Shobha: "So many illnesses come because of the worries. Tension, mental tension - you can't sleep very well with the tension. Then, when that will pass, it will lead to illness, won't it?" She goes onto suggest that Asian women in Britain look much older than British women, because, she feels, the latter have fewer worries.

Rani connects mental and physical ill-health with worries: "When you are worrying, then you are mentally ill, you feel physically ill too. You have pain in the chest, headache - all these kind of things." It is Naseem who links worries closely with depression, believing that they are separate, but that they are, "the worst cause for illness. Nothing can cause you more illness than these two things." The worries that the women have, about their personal circumstances, their domestic responsibilities and their families and friends far away, all weigh very heavily on them, and they feel that these worries do result in ill-health, both mental exhaustion and physical pain.

Germs and Viruses

All the informants acknowledge that some episodes of ill-health are caused by external agents, commonly known as germs. Naseem says: "Disease is caused by some germs, and that can be only physical ... throat infections, chest infections and any other kind of infections in the body." Rani agrees: "There are many illnesses caused by the germs. The 'flu - one person can catch the 'flu from the other ... TB is a very contagious disease which is spread out due to the germs ... Also smallpox and the measles."

The capacity of germs to cause illness is related to the body's resistance: "If you are healthy, and if you have got a good immunity, then you will be less attacked by the germs. Then if you are a weak person, you will be more attacked by the germs and quickly you will catch the disease from another person" (Tasneem). Rani also mentions the body's inbuilt resistance to outside attack: "We have some germs that keep us healthy" (Rani), and Naseem explains that she means anti-bodies. Naseem goes into more detail: "You have got some natural resistance to germs and viruses if your anti-bodies are strong, and then the things can get better quickly if you are strong and healthy ... You must be very strong to fight with viruses." Naseem has heard of viruses, which she describes as, "Some sort of germ which attack you, where the anti-biotics can't help you. It's your body which resists them and can cure them."

In the life-story interviews, most of the women mention fever and 'flu as common illnesses which are sometimes caused by germs. Some talk of specific instances of germs causing ill-health: Sufiya, for example, says of smallpox: "My cousin's sister's daughters had it first, and they died. We went to the funeral and must have caught it there." Tasneem speaks of a tuberculosis germ which infected her son's hand after he had been bitten by an ass in Pakistan. The infection was not diagnosed for some time, despite the attention of health service doctors, a Harley Street specialist, and finally an American specialist after a skin sample had been flown to New York. Tasneem thinks that the family's health problems may have resulted from exposure to this germ, and that it particularly affected her: "I was ill also - perhaps that [the TB germ] caused all my trouble" (Tasneem). (Her story is considered in full in the health services section).

Some of the informants emphasise the importance of keeping the body's resistance high against invading germs, and the best way of doing this is seen to be by keeping everything clean and pure. There is a clear link here between religious beliefs and practices and maintaining good health, for the women's religions all demand strict cleanliness and purity, and they believe that this, in turn, leads to good health: "Germs are the cause of illness, and to avoid the germs, cleanliness is the best thing ... Cleanliness and freshness [of food]" (Rani).

Fate and God's will are seen to largely determine who gets which germ, when and where, although the informants do allow that the body's resistance can be helped to withstand some infections (see above). Only Naseem has heard of viruses - the other women who were asked said that they had no knowledge of them. Overall, germs are seen to be an important cause of physical illnesses and diseases, and they are linked with the issues of temperature, religion and weight which are pivotal concepts for these informants and are considered in detail, in the culture section.

Heredity

The idea of the possible inheritance of ill-health is not something the informants care to dwell upon. Naseem told me, off tape, that there is a great shame in their community attached to families who have inheritable conditions because of their affect on the marriageability of children, and that any families with such diseases or illnesses go to great lengths to hide them. Naseem gave the example of Geeta, whose daughter is suspected of suffering from some sort of fits or epilepsy, but Geeta made no mention of this and the daughter is rarely seen.

Rani's husband made his only serious interjection during Rani's discussion of heredity. He began to tell of a condition that is present in Rani's family, tuberculosis of the glands, which supposedly caused the death of her brother. At this point, Rani swiftly silenced him, adding, "It is not necessary that because the parent has got some illness, that the children should get it necessarily, but there are some chances."

There are several indications in the life-story interviews that the informants do believe that certain illnesses and diseases "run in the family". Conditions which have no stigma, such as heart disease, TB, diabetes, high blood pressure, rheumatism and asthma are suggested. Rani, Dalee and Baji say that someone in their family has, "sugar in the urine", or sugar diabetes, with Dalee adding that, "My father's whole family was diabetic, so they were careful about the sugar ... ate special things." Sufiya's son's thalassaemia is hereditary (see chapter three), but Sufiya does not necessarily believe it: "They [the doctors] were asking me whether or not anyone in the family has got this trouble, but this is the first child to have it. Nobody else." Thus it would seem that heredity is seen as an important cause of ill-health, but that it is hidden if the conditions are visible or could affect the family's social standing. As with the Afro-Caribbean informants, there is a tendency to see heredity as important, but not in relation to one's own family.

Other Causes of Ill-Health

The environment is seen to be an important cause of ill-health, particularly through the influence of the weather, housing conditions and just by being in Britain rather than anywhere else. These factors are considered in the living in Britain section. Other important causes of ill-health are also dealt with elsewhere: weight, temperature and food, for example, (see culture section). In general, this section on the causes of ill-health is inextricably linked to many of the other sections, particularly those concerning living in Britain, cultural and personal inheritance and the severity of ill-health. Throughout the interviews, most of the informants profess no knowledge of the causes of episodes of ill-health, but there are many instances where they guess at causes while telling stories about the conditions and their experiences of them. Often of greater concern than the origin of a condition is the alleviation of its symptoms, and here the influence of fate, religion and culture play important roles. The context of each event is also important. The informants are affected by recent events and discussions and these can direct their answers in particular ways. An understanding of the context of what they say is, therefore, crucial.

The Severity of Ill-Health

Incurable illnesses/diseases

All the informants are afraid of getting some kind of serious complaint: "I am afraid of getting the nervous breakdown. That sometimes the tension gets so bad that you can't sleep all night" (Naseem); "Everybody is scared of losing any part of the body. We are always praying to God that he should keep our sight and that we should keep our hands and feet" (Rani); "There are many illnesses which we are afraid of, like paralysis, blindness, stroke, cancer ... We always pray that God should save us from all of these illnesses" (Tasneem); and "I am scared of being paralysed ... that is the worst thing which can happen. I am afraid of having to depend on other people" (Shobha). The women are particularly affected in their answers by their own recent experiences. Naseem, Rani and Tasneem are all close friends of Dalee, and their answers reflect their shocked reaction to her latest stroke which has left her partially paralysed and, temporarily, they hope, blind. Similarly, Shobha's mother and father have recently died of strokes, having been paralysed for some time and being totally dependent on one of Shobha's brothers. These examples emphasise that the context of people's answers is crucial to an understanding of them.

Most of the women believe that there are incurable illnesses and/or diseases. Naseem has suffered all her life with coeliac disease and she hopes that they will find a cure eventually, although all the doctors can do now is to advise her not to eat any flour. She says, hopefully, "In this advanced scientific age, I don't think that any illness is incurable except cancer, but for cancer too they are finding a cure ... It's just a matter of finding the cause ... I think that it can be cured, easily, especially those illnesses where surgery is needed. Those are quite curable, more than the other illnesses when there is some mental cause also" (Naseem). The acceptance of what happens to her comes through here, as does her faith in western medicine.

Many of the informants cite cancer as an incurable disease, but, like Naseem, they reveal great faith in western medicine and doctors: "I'm not sure [about the cause of cancer]. Sometimes they say people who smoke too much can get lung cancer, and some people get lung cancer without even smoking, so I don't really know what causes the cancer. The doctors only know who are doing the research" (Tasneem). The context is again important for Rani's answer. She has faith in doctors, but she does not believe that they can cure cancer because, she says, even one of the richest men in the world, the Shah of Iran, died of it: "If money could've done something, he would have been cured" (Rani).

Several other conditions are thought to be incurable. Sufiya, for example, says of smallpox: "There is no proper cure. Nothing can stop it until the body is covered, and then it needs time to recover." Rani, Dalee and Baji, whose husbands have sugar diabetes, see that as incurable, although they are not too worried as it can be controlled with, "proper food" (Baji). It would seem that Sufiya has not been told that her son's thalassaemia is incurable at present, as she says she hopes he will, "grow out of it", or at least put on sufficient weight to allow doctors to operate on his hole in the heart. Dalee seems to accept that her ill-health is incurable. She says her disease is called "SLE", but she has no knowledge of what these letters stand for or what the disease actually is. It is a condition that affects the nervous system. Dalee's health problems are a constant worry to her, and she says that she cannot see any future for herself: "I just see that one day I am going to die. I just think that" (Dalee).

The question of whether or not the informants believe that any illnesses or diseases are inevitable, proved hard to translate. Instead of inevitable conditions, the women remember illnesses and diseases which were quite common when they or their grandparents were children, but which are rarely heard of nowadays. They speak of such things as malnutrition, tuberculosis, smallpox and the plague. Their reason for the disappearance of these conditions is summed up by Rani, who says, "Science and medicine are very advanced now and there are many, many illnesses that the doctors have got control of."

Serious Illnesses/Diseases

Eight of the informants claim that they have never been seriously ill (Naseem, Taresh, Syeda, Sufiya, Geeta, Farah, Rajinda and Farida). Naseem claims this despite suffering constantly from coeliac disease. Dalee readily admits that she has been, and still is, seriously ill. She developed rheumatoid arthritis after the birth of her second child, and was advised not to have any more children. Unfortunately, she had two more pregnancies, one of which ended in a miscarriage, and another which went to the full term and left Dalee extremely weak. "Since then," she says, "the health is no good. In 1976, I had a stroke due to high blood pressure. Since then, I am getting down, down, down" (Dalee).

The first stroke left Dalee paralysed down one side, and she has been virtually house-bound since then. In 1980, she had another stroke, this time affecting her voice and necessitating many visits to hospital for speech therapy. "Now," she says, "I am all right, but sometimes I faint." A week before the life-story interview, Dalee had slipped on ice getting out of a car, had fallen heavily and broke her arm, further constraining her mobility. As indicated above, just before I returned to the women to ask them the focused questions, Dalee had had another stroke which increased her paralysis and left her blind. The doctors are unsure as to whether or not the blindness is temporary.

Some of the other women consider that they have also been seriously ill: Rani had a gall-bladder operation; Tasneem suffered from tuberculosis; Shobha had anaemia and felt unable to eat properly for several months; Baji lost a lot of blood when she had heavy periods and eventually had a hysterectomy; and Reena is worried about her severe headaches and the cataract operation she is due to have. The important details of these episodes are recorded in the health services section.

Psychological Influences on Health

Although there is not a specific word in Urdu which sums up the feeling of depression, most of the women understand the term. For many, depression is almost indistinguishable from loneliness, and along with worries, it is thought to have clear effects on health. For these informants, loneliness and depression are part of everyday life, and bring back memories of past times abroad. Shobha sums up many of the women's feelings about loneliness: "It can cause a lot of illnesses. You feel depressed, you feel unhappy. Since I lost my parents, I feel like this ... I feel very depressed sometimes, especially when I am alone ... Now I feel lonely and that makes me feel ill and depressed sometimes."

Rani compares life in Britain with life in Pakistan, and speculates on the effects of loneliness: "Loneliness is the worst thing which can cause illness. If you are sitting on your own, you are all the time thinking about things. You have nobody to talk to. If you are with someone, you are speaking, you are just telling what is in your heart and so you don't feel ill, you feel happy. But if you are alone, then you will always feel sick. In our country, people are meeting each other all the time and they are coming and asking how you are and that helps a lot with your health." She continues to say that the people who go to work are best off because they can go out and meet people, "but the ladies who are sitting alone in the house, it is bad for their health if they are alone all the time" (Rani). For Tasneem, the loneliness of life in Britain is compared with a prison: "Loneliness is the worst thing a person can have. It can cause a lot of illnesses. When the person is sent to the gaol ... the only thing he lacks is the company. There are two parts to this thing about health. The first part is to eat good food and the second is to talk to each other. You need good food and company to keep you healthy."

Although some of the informants do meet regularly at the local club, and many visit each other in their homes, this is not enough to alleviate the overwhelming feeling of loneliness they have. They all admit to missing friends and relatives, and particularly miss being able to meet people they know if they leave their homes. In Britain, they may be alone for many hours while other members of their families are at work or school, and this time leads to boredom and nostalgia for "home".

For some of the informants, loneliness and depression are intricately connected, with loneliness causing depression and depression leading to more loneliness in a frustrating cycle: "I used to be very depressed, missing my parents and sister. I still do miss them" (Naseem); "We feel depressed when we think of our parents and so on in Pakistan, and sometimes we cry when we miss them and when we see there is no-one around here close to us" (Taresh); "We are all depressed here, missing our parents" (Syeda); "My husband goes to work all day, my son goes to college, and Farida goes up to sleep, so I am all on my own. I can't sleep during the day, so I do feel depressed" (Farah); "I miss my past times in India. I miss my friends, my college ... Now I am just sitting here, doing nothing, missing all those times" (Farida).

For some of the informants, these feelings of desolation and loneliness are also expressed in a desire to return to their countries of birth, but this is not true of many. Farida wants to return, but her parents will not let her because they intend to bring over the entire family. Farah hopes that she will, "get used to it, in time." Dalee would like to return, but thinks that she will not be able to because of her unstable health and need for constant attention. Her recent attempt to visit Pakistan led to another stroke. Most of the others express fond memories of their past homes, but few say categorically that they would like to return. As women, they feel that their duty is to their husbands and children, and since their family homes are in Britain, and many of their children are British, they realise they will never return.

Some of the informants are depressed for reasons other than loneliness. Naseem and Tasneem are depressed because of their ill-health. For Naseem, it is her back injury which adds to her loneliness: "I am feeling depressed because I can't walk much because of my back. I can't get out. I'm on my own in the house." Tasneem's husband is concerned about Tasneem's health, and, she says, "Sometimes I feel depressed for nothing. My husband takes me out somewhere, so that I might feel better. He is also scared that I might be ill again" (Tasneem). She also believes that worrying about relatives abroad and not being able to get in touch with them can lead to depression an ill-health.

Several of the informants claim never to get depressed, usually because of their strong religious beliefs: "I keep myself very busy and I pray to God all the time, and if you pray to God, you never feel depressed" (Baji); "I believe in God, I never get depressed" (Rani). Dalee is another who claims that she never gets depressed, yet during the interview, she gave several indications that she is depressed. She says, "I am very happy at home myself, I put on the TV, sometimes I watch it," but she goes on to say, "All I can see is that one day I am going to die. I just think that" (Dalee).

Shobha recalls that she was depressed for a short time when her husband wanted his parents to live with them, and although she was given tranquilizers, she says, "I didn't take many - only valium. It didn't help if I had tranquilizers too much, it's not good for my health ... So, better than take valium, I used to go shopping, to friends, for a walk" (Shobha). For Sufiya, the only cause of her depression is her son's illness.

For Rajinda and Reena, depression is a more constant companion. Rajinda's depression and loneliness are caused by bereavement. Her husband was shot, accidently, at his brother's wedding, and then a few months later, their only child died. Rajinda says, "I am not ill, but I feel upset sometimes. It's the pressure of it ... The worry for me. I get headaches and pains and aches in the body." Rajinda also gets anxious and nervous if anyone calls on her to tell her of any news. Similarly, Reena also gets headaches and feelings of anxiety. She thinks the headaches may arise from her cataracts, but she also speaks of her family worries concerning her son-in-law's inability to enter Britain, and adds, "The people over here talk a lot, saying the husband doesn't want to come over ... I worry a lot ... The people, they all talk about each other a lot, and it puts pressure on us, causes the worry" (Reena).

There are clear and close links between these views on depression and those on the influence of worries on health. Rani says, "When you are worrying, when you are mentally ill, you feel physically ill too. You have pain in the chest, headache - all these kind of things." It is, however, Naseem who makes the most explicit links between worries, depression and loneliness: "Depression and worry can cause more illnesses than any other thing. If you are depressed, tensed up, you will get so many illnesses where the doctor will never find out why they are caused. Your stomach may get upset, your blood pressure will rise, you won't be able to sleep with depression ... Depression and worry are the worst cause for illness. Nothing can cause you more illness that these two things ... Most of the people in Britain and the world, I think they are ill because they are depressed ... I sometimes think that I am more depressed than ill" (Naseem).

The influence of tiredness on health is insignificant when compared with the perceived effects of loneliness and depression on the informants. Some do concede that tiredness can be a factor in ill-health. Few of the women work, and so they do not feel as tired as the women of Afro-Caribbean descent. Sufiya concedes that having to tend her son constantly, and to administer his overnight injections tires her out and that she consequently feels ill. For some, tiredness is a feeling tht indicates that a person might be unwell: "I felt a bit weak. First of all I thought it was too much work ... perhaps I was exhausted, but then they found out I had high blood pressure" (Tasneem); "It is mostly due to the tiredness that you feel very ill" (Naseem); "If you are over tired, if you are tensed up, you will feel ill" (Rani).

Shock is another psychological effect which the informants feel can impinge on ill-health. It is related to their feelings of isolation and loneliness, and usually occurs when bad news arrives suddenly from abroad. Rani remembers how she felt when she heard her parents were dead: "My blood pressure went up and I felt a lot of pain in the body and

I wasn't feeling myself for a long time. I was crying all the time and I felt the loss very much indeed. It was shock that gave me the illness." Rajinda worries in case news might come to her like it did when her husband was killed: "I'm very nervous if I hear any news or if somebody comes suddenly. I just start shaking."

Tasneem recalls a story about her brother which links the effects of shock, religion and death: "We came to Pakistan at the partition time and the grandfather died, and my elder brother felt the shock of losing him very much. He started getting a temperature and fell ill ... Our people believe in spirits, and sometimes my mother felt he had some shadows, some possession, so they used to take him to the priests and all ... Sometimes they took him to the hospital too, but he still died, aged ten years. They took him mostly to the other places, rather than the medical treatment" (Tasneem).

The effects of shock are also clearly exhibited in the reactions of Naseem and Tasneem to the sudden news of Dalee's stroke. Although she is always unwell, the suddenness of the arrival of the stroke after a gap of four years since the last is made worse by the fact that Dalee was supposed to be visiting Pakistan the day after it happened. The suddenness frightened Naseem and Tasneem: "Sudden news can be a terrible shock. You feel very ill. Like this lady [Dalee], when we heard, all of us were really shocked and we felt very ill" (Taneem); and "I cried all night. I was ill, just thinking how she is" (Naseem).

The effects of such things as depression, loneliness, shock, tiredness and worries on the informants' lives are thus enormous. Depression, loneliness and worries in particular are seen to be crucial in causing or exacerbating feelings of ill-health, and they are perceived to affect both physical and mental health. Loneliness is an especially pervasive problem for these women, isolated as they are from their families and friends, and their difficulties are compounded by the coldness of the climate in Britain and the hostility of the white population. Despite feelings of depression and loneliness, the women accept that life has to go on, and they concentrate on coping with day-to-day worries and illnesses. The next section outlines some of the ways in which these informants cope with episodes of ill-health.

Cultural and Personal Heritage

"Culture" here is loosely defined as those ideas and attitudes which are drawn from a person's heritage and which have some influence on life-style and behaviour and, ultimately, health.

Remedies

Home remedies are one outcome of people's attempts to cope with episodes of ill-health. The degree to which they are used depends upon their presence in each individual's personal, family and cultural group, their perceived efficacy and upon the faith placed on modern medicine and its techniques. In this group of women of Asian descent, the tendency is to rely on modern medicine rather than any other ways of coping with ill-health. A few speak of remedies they can remember being used when they were children, but very few use any of these now. Many of these informants come from wealthy families, and hold hakims, the traditioal practitioners of herbal medicines, in low esteem. Consequently, they have not used and would not use herbal or home preparations, except as a last resort. Hakims are viewed as the doctors for the very poor of the sub-continent, who are paid only for their prescriptions. The wealthy of the sub-continent, they say, rely on western medicine, and so the majority of these informants have great faith in their western-trained GPs and local hospitals.

Naseem, Tasneem, Reena, Rajinda and Taresh mention their families using hakims or herbal preparations many years ago. Herbal teas seem to be a common family remedy; otherwise hakims were used only when all other methods of health care had failed. Reena recalls: "If we used to have anything wrong, our parents used to give us some herbs, boil some herbs to give us, and that used to help." Rajinda and Naseem remember using a mixture of herbs called, "banakshaa": "You boil the herbs up and drink it and that was very good for coughs and colds. My grandmother and mother talked about it. The hakims used to sell this. The people would keep herbs in the house and would drink it when everybody had coughs and colds. It is helpful for the asthma, too" (Rajinda). Naseem also used to have a herbal mixture for her stomach, which is now available in this country under the label, "fibogel".

Several of the women agree with Sufiya when she says, "They might have had some special things, but I can't remember." Others can recall a few preparations such as a mixture of almond powders and milk and apple jam (Farah); anadin for headaches (Rani); panadol and lemon tea for 'flu (Taresh); benelyn syrup and hot drinks for 'flu (Sufiya), and boiling water with or without lemon juice, "for the tummy and the headache" (Rajinda). Baji recalls that her grandmother would not allow her to drink too much tea: "She said tea is like a drug and you will get addicted to it", so Baji always had to drink milk.

Only one of the women expresses a clear preference for one type of drug. Rajinda says, "Tablets and capsules are easy to swallow. I can't drink the mixture or take the powders because you can taste it. My husband used to force me to take it and afterwards he gave me sugar." Most of the women seem not to mind in what form a drug comes, and the rest will take medicine or tablets. Some indicate that they prefer injections where these are posssible, because they have had iron injections which have cleared up their anaemia faster than any other sort of drugs (Naseem, Geeta and Shobha), and they have become accustomed to having injections when they travel to India or Pakistan. Their lack of faith in medicines and preference for tablets may come from their reluctance to rely on "poor people's" remedies, but willingness to trust western drugs.

Religion

Only Farida and Dalee say that they are not very religious - all of the other informants are very faithful to their religions and rely on them a great deal for peace and comfort. Seven are Muslims (Naseem, Taresh, Syeda, Rani, Tasneem, Sufiya and Dalee); four are Sikhs (Shobha, Baji, Rajinda and Reena); and three are Hindus (Farah, Farida and Geeta). The Sikhs and Hindus pray outside the home, the Hindus in a temple, and the Sikhs at Gurdwara (temple), and both seem to pray at least once a day. The Muslim women tend not to go outside to pray, but most pray frequently at home. Rani, for example, prays five times a day, and she did so both times I was present, complaining at one stage that the focused questions had caused her to miss a prayer time. The Muslim prayers are energetic: "I do exercise enough because of our prayer. You have to exercise, bending down, standing up, bowing. Five times a day" (Rani). Naseem's back injury means that she connot manage this level of activity, and Sufiya finds that she does not have time for it because of her constant caring for her son.

Religious beliefs and faith in God give the women a great sense of peace and contentment, and they help to ease the burden of worries, depression and loneliness: "Prayer helps very much, even when you are very depressed. It would help more than the tranquilizers" (Naseem); "I go to Gurdwara very often. It helps and it makes me feel better" (Shobha); "I pray to God all the time, and if you pray to God, you never feel depressed. I have never worried in my life" (Baji); "I feel contentment in the heart when I pray" (Taresh); "I am religious. I don't believe in fortune tellers. I only believe in one God. It helps me. I don't believe in spells and things. I am not superstitious. Just pray to God and not depend on anybody else" (Reena); "You are more peaceful when you are praying to God and more relaxed. It eases the worries" (Tasneem).

For Rajinda, it is faith which has finally enabled her to cope with the deaths of her husband and child, and the blame placed on her by her husband's family: "When my husband and daughter died, I lost my confidence even in God, and I said, 'I am not going to Gurdwara or say any prayers.' I used to talk and say things because I lost my faith ... I used to say, 'God hasn't done fair to me, so I don't believe in Him.' So the in-laws started making trouble and I couldn't go anywhere but the Gurdwara. Since then, I am feeling better. It is the most helpful thing. God is the best to you - nobody else is ... It is your belief which keeps you going. It is only God who is helping me at the moment. No companion have I got" (Rajinda).

Religious beliefs do not only help the women overcome, or at least cope with the pervasive feelings of depression and loneliness, but they also influence health more directly: "Religion helps a lot. When my child was ill, my mother-in-law prayed a lot and we gave charity to the poor and sometimes I think that may be my child is getting better due to the prayers rather than the medicine" (Sufiya); "Prayers are more helpful than the medicine" (Geeta); "Those who believe in God and pray to God, they must be certainly healthier than the others, mentally and physically

... Prayers do help, along with the medicines, but I don't think that a person who is a religious person can never be ill ... But religious people are mentally peaceful I am sure" (Naseem).

Cleanliness and purity are concepts that are related to the religious views of the informants. Rani in particular stresses the influence of religion on cleanliness and, ultimately, health: "The things which are contained in the religion, they are based on the health." She thinks particularly of the exercises of bending and stretching involved in prayer, and, she says, "We wash ourselves five times - that keeps you clean ... You fast - one months fast - that also clarifies all things in your body ... it keeps your weight normal, so it keeps you healthy" (Rani). Purity is seen to be important through many of the informants' references to the need for "pure" food to remain in good health, and also a comment made by Sufiya about fits from which her son suffers: "By a big clot in his head, caused by the heart trouble - it doesn't purify the blood properly and it doesn't circulate properly" (Sufiya).

In sum, the majority of the informants' lives are influenced enormously, if not controlled by, the tenets of their religions. For some, this means avoiding certain foods, originally for health reasons, but now out of principle or religious law. Muslims, for example, do not eat pork, and Hindus are not supposed to eat meat, although they are starting to do so in Britain (see below). For others, it means that their lives are organised around the time to pray or to go to the place of worship. Above all of these influences in everyday life, religious beliefs outline the ways to cope with such events as shocks or episodes of ill-health, and give the women the strength to deal with the depression and loneliness from which they suffer. Their faith affects their mental and physical health, giving strength and peacefulness against all the unpleasantnesses they have to face. In short, religion is a crucial, pivotal concept in an understanding of the lives of these informants and their states of health.

Food

All of the informants believe that food has an important role in the maintenance of good health. Many of them have adopted some western dishes because they say that their children tend to prefer them: things such as beefburgers, minced meat and fish fingers; but many also still cook traditional dishes for their husbands and themselves. They are lucky in their area to have access to a number of shops selling Asian produce at reasonable prices, and the council has also employed a Asian dietician to advise the women on what foods are nutritious and how they should be cooked. Contrary to some of the advice which comes from the DHSS, the dietician spends much of her time emphasising the value of traditional Asian food, and describing to the women the most advantageous ways to prepare it.

Two of the women remark that the food in Britain is better than that found in India because it is perceived to be, "Clean and pure" (Syeda and Rani). Baji, however, complains that, "The meat in this country is not fresh, and frozen meat is not very good for health. In our country [India], you go straight to the butcher and get fresh meat, but in this country, the meat is very stale." Rani agrees: "With cleanliness, we must have pure food, nutritious food: vegetables, milk and all these things keep healthy. Freshness and cleanliness ... I like fresh food better than the frozen ... fresh food is better." Farah's diet has changed since her family arrived in Britain: "We never used to eat meat before in India, but now my husband makes [cooks] chicken or meat, so he forces the children to eat it because this is a cold country." Farah's husband feels the need to offset the coldness of Britain with a "hot" food: meat. There are links here with the beliefs about "hot" and "cold" and the need to balance these in the body explored below.

Two of the informants declare outright that they do not eat meat: "It's not that it is bad for health, but according to our religion, our God won't allow us to eat meat" (Geeta); and Baji, who says that eating meat is cruel to animals, and that, "Fresh fruit and vegetables are better than meat ... Even the doctors say you should eat fresh fruit and vegetables!" Baji made this statement after she discovered that I do not eat meat. Unlike Geeta, Baji does not abstain from meat for religious reasons, but because she dislikes it.

A lot of the informants emphasise that dairy products are important for good health, and only Farida mentions not drinking milk. Of dairy foods, they say: "We used pure ghee [clarified butter], milk and butter to keep ourselves healthy" (Reena); "Because we were farmers, we had fresh milk, pure butter and vegetables ... this kind of things we used to keep in our house to keep us healthy" (Tasneem); "We never used any [remedies], just milk and fruit" (Geeta); "We never used medicine, but we took lots of pure milk, butter and yoghurt. Because we had cows in our house, we could have all these things fresh" (Baji); "Butter is very good for health - it gives energy. Milk is good as well, fresh milk" (Reena). With opinions as strong as these, it is not really surprising that the rickets campaign's attempts to persuade Asians to replace butter with margarine have largely failed. Some of the informants do use margarine rather than butter, but the majority do not believe that margarine could be better for them than butter because their experience suggests the superiority of butter.

Three of the women complain that they find it difficult to digest food in Britain. For Naseem, this is because she has coeliac disease, and she finds it difficult to eat suitable foods, particularly as her traditional staple, chapattis, are normally made of gluten-rich wheat flour. The other two do not have a physical illness, but they say they suffer from digestion difficulties: "In India ... we just digest it ... Perhaps it was the heat ... We used to walk around a lot too ... I was not fat over there, and we used to eat fried food, but in this country, we feel we can't digest the fried food ... It just stays in the stomach ... If I eat fried chapattis now, here, I get indigestion and headache, always" (Rajinda); and, "In India, I used to eat two big chapattis made of cornflour and two made of wheat flour, but over here, I can hardly eat one and a half. I can't digest very much food" (Reena).

Certain foods are perceived to cause or help to cure ill-health. As indicated above, dairy produce and fresh fruit and vegetables are thought to keep the body healthy. Other foods are perceived to cause or exacerbate ill-health. Rajinda says, for example, "Once I had an allergy on my body - an itchy rash. I used to drink a lot of tea, and that's what caused the itching." Shobha remembers having chickenpox as a child, and she says, "We were careful when cooking the curries. It is thought that the fried onion is harmful for the chickenpox. I avoided that, also meat, eggs, things like that. We think that smallpox and chickenpox are due to the anger of a Goddess and we shouldn't annoy that Goddess. If we eat meat and egg, it will get worse." Religious beliefs are thus shown again to be crucial. Rani and Baji also mention that eating any food is dangerous when a person is suffering from typhoid.

A few of the remedies for ill-health mentioned above are composed of food. There are some others reported by the informants: "Cauliflower, they say it gives you too much wind in the tummy, and they used to put a lot of ginger in it for the remedy of that" (Tasneem); and, "My mother thought ginger and garlic were very good for aches and pains ... In this country, once a week, I used to fry some onion, ginger and garlic and eat it with tomatoes, salt and pepper" (Rajinda). Others just emphasise the importance of, "a very balanced diet ... If we eat the proper food, then only will we be able to do certain things" (Rani); and, "I think if we can eat good food and stay healthy, in that way we will save money ... Food is the most important thing for your health. You should spend more on the food than on any other thing in the house ... You can get good immunity by eating good food" (Taneem).

Food is thus perceived to be another crucial variable in the maintenance of good health by most of the informants who can choose between a wide variety of traditional and modern foods. Supplementary to this, the concepts of "hot" and "cold" which are very important to many of the informants, are linked to the importance of food. In many cases, the notion of balance is thought to be very important, either the balance of the diet, or the balance of hot and cold forces within the diet. This will now be examined more fully.

Temperature and "Hot" and "Cold"

The informants believe, largely, in the importance of balance in the body. This is usually expressed in terms of balancing heat and cold, and so a person's temperature is seen to be an important aspect of their health. A "normal" temperature signals health, and any deviation from this is seen to be indicative of some sort of ill-health. The concern about a person being hot or cold has been passed down to the informants by their parents and grandparents, but the beliefs are being rapidly eroded by westernization. Western medicine and thought ignores the old ways handed down to the informants, and so many of them are now skeptical of the value of traditional ideas. Nevertheless, the concepts of hot and cold are rooted also in their own experiences, and the influence of some of these beliefs has persisted, affecting the informants' attitudes to ill-health and its treatment. The focused questions were directed specifically at getting the informants to talk about these beliefs, although there had been many indications of their importance from the life-story interviews.

There are many instances where the informants say that they, or their relatives, had a temperature and were, therefore, ill. Rajinda, Baji and Rani remember a major symptom of typhoid being a high temperature; Sufiya's son had a very high temperature before he had a fit; Rajinda's daughter, "got a high temperature and chikenpox" before her death; Tasneem, "Had the 'flu and the temperature", which turned into pheumonia and tuberculosis; and Reena recalls that her headaches are, "like a burning sensation in my head." Fever, the most common sort of ill-health reported by the informants, is also determined by the effect it has on a person's temperature. The proverb, "Feed a cold; starve a fever" is a well-known English lay belief associated with temperature (see Helman, 1976).

Some illnesses or diseases are defined by the informants to be "hot" or "cold", and balance is restored in the body by taking hot or cold foods to cancel out the excess . A hot temperature, for example, is seen by all the informants as an obvious indication that someone is ill, and so Shobha suggests using, "cold things to bring it down - cold drinks or something." Rani concurs, "If you get a high temperature, then you have to use cold compresses. With the heat, you help with the cold things." Measles is thought to be, "a very hot disease. It can make the children very ill, the temperature is very high", and consequently, "they can't eat chicken, meat, eggs and so on because they are very hot foods" (Naseem). Rani talks about jaundice and burning in the urine to be very hot conditions, and she explains the notion of balance: "You have to get a balance in the bile of the body - the hot things cause you bile and heat in the body and then it upsets your stomach ... so to balance them you have to take some cold things."

Hot foods and drinks can have bad effects. "They used to think that egg, chicken, dried fruit are very hot, so you shouldn't eat very much of them because they will raise your blood pressure or make you bleed too much" (Naseem). Also, "tea and coffee is [sic] very hot. It affects your stomach, it upsets your stomach" (Naseem). Some foods such as karela (an Asian vegetable) "can give you a little bit heart-burning ... because it is hot" (Naseem); "Nuts and things like that give you heat in the stomach or chest ... the hot food can cause jaundice" (Rani); "Spices and hot foods can cause ulcers in the stomach" (Shobha); and, "Certain spices which we think are very hot, they can upset your stomach and they upset your head ... Pickles, they are said to give you the sore throat ... Coffee and tea we think are very hot drinks and it upsets your stomach" (Tasneem).

These hot foods can be balanced by cold foods, but cold foods in excess can also cause ill-effects. "There are certain foods that they think are cold, like fruit, vegetables, carrots etc, and these are good for your health. Also yoghurt and orange juice are cold. Sometimes too much of the cold foods will give you headaches, but cold things, they are good for your health and hot food is not very good" (Naseem). "Mango and melon ... orange juice or oranges and lemons are considered to be cold" (Rani). Tasneem remembers some advice: "They used to say that oranges were very cold, so don't eat oranges in cold weather, they will give you headache."

Too many cold foods or drinks can also have very serious side-effects: "You can get sort of asthma trouble with the cold things like ice-cream, cold drinks in winter" (Shobha); "My cousin died in Saudi Arabia - he was fasting for the whole day ... Ramadan, and he drank the cold water and died instantly" (Naseem); "If you come from outside in a hot climate and at once drink something very cold, like lemon or orange juice with some ice ... sometimes it can cause pneumonia" (Rani). Rani gives her own advice as to how to overcome this: "If you go in the very hot climate, the sunshine, you sometimes get a headache. Then if you drink something, you will feel better, but you shouldn't drink straight away, you should sit for a while and rest."

An important idea emerges about Western drugs. Naseem explains that she thinks Asian people, "think the English medicines are hot - in the way that they give more side-effects ... Like sometimes if you have anti-biotics, it makes you feel very drowsy and sleepy ... they think this is a sort of heat ... They think the hakims or the homeopathic medicine is cold. It has got no side-effects, only good effects."

Tasneem concurs: "In our country, they think that herbal treatment is cool and soothing, there are no side-effects, but the medicines, they are hot, they are not very good, they can give them side-effects due to the chemicals in them. Herbs, on the other hand, they are natural things. I mean, even if they don't give you good effects, they won't give you any bad effects!" Geeta actually practises this: "He [the doctor] said I needed the iron tablets ... He told me to take three tablets a day, but I am taking only one. I feel too hot with three - like hot flushes. They don't agree with me." Shobha and Rajinda also report that they do not take the prescribed amount of their drugs, and the influence of ideas about hot and cold may be an important reason for some non-compliance.

There seems to be a contradiction here between what these women say about herbal treatments and their general feelings towards hakims expressed earlier. Naseem and Tasneem are here referring to older Asian people who still follow the old ways in the sub-continent, where medicines may be scarce and herbal treatments more easily available and trusted. They are also referring to a deeply held belief about western drugs which is being eroded in Britain and which they no longer adhere to. Having been westernised, Tasneem and Naseem are now skeptical of herbal treatments and make derrogatory comments about hakims, but Geeta, who is older and much less westernised, still clings to the traditional fear of "hot" western drugs.

Although the more westernised women are skeptical about some of the old beliefs concerning hot and cold, they can see some justifications for using them: "There is a lot of truth in these old ideas. I mean, it was due to their experience they found out these things. Even on TV, they say that the homeopathic treatment is better that the English treatment" (Tasneem); "They can't eat chicken, meat, eggs and so on because these are very hot foods ... In a way they are right - eggs have too much cholesterol. They are right in some way. They can't tell why they are saying it, the old ladies say it, so may be they knew what the side-effects were. They learned it by their experience and they were right" (Naseem). There is also agreement in old and new beliefs that tea and coffee are not good for you: the old view being that they are "hot", that they can damage the stomach and that they are so dry they will prevent sleep; the modern view being that caffeine in tea and coffee can damage the stomach lining, and cause insomnia.

The issue of temperature is, therefore, important for these informants. It connects clearly with beliefs about food, and provides many ways for the informants to cope with and understand episodes of ill-health. Heat and cold are important markers of ill-health, and their balance is a recognised method of curing conditions, or at least alleviating their symptoms. These views persist despite the tendency of western medicine to ignore them, but some of the informants manage to employ both traditional and modern beliefs in their methods of health care.

Miscellaneous factors

Another example of the clash between traditional and modern views comes over the issue of weight. This was often an important talking point for the women after the interview had finished. Syeda explains the traditional view through her worries about a daughter: "Three of them [children] are quite healthy, but the eldest one is a bit slim. She is healthy, but her structure is quite small. Our people think that if they are slim, they are not healthy. Fat people are said to be healthier than slim" (Syeda). Syeda also exhibits the influence of western ideas, as she continues, "I think the slim are more active, strong and healthy. Fat people look healthy, but they aren't."

In the life-story interviews, several of the women showed that they still adhered to the old belief that to be fat is healthy and to be slim is unhealthy. Dalee says of her husband, "He is all right ... Slim, but healthy"; Naseem says of her sons: "One is very healthy, very tall and he eats very well. The other one is small and he doesn't eat very much at all and I am worried about him"; and Dalee says of her children: "The eldest child is healthier than the other - the small one is a bit slim, and the older is fatter and healthier, but now the little one is also getting fat, so I am happy." Tasneem mentions that one of her children was very small and ill at birth, but that, "she began to put on weight, and she got better." Sufiya hopes that her thalassaemia-suffering son will put on weight because it is seen to be an indication of getting well again.

The westernization evident in much of the informants' lives is exhibited in some of their statements about weight. As indicated by Syeda, there is some movement over to the western views that, "slim is best", or that average weight is good: "They think in this country that slim people are healthier than fat people, but I don't know, sometimes the slim people are also ill ... In our community, they think fat people are healthiest ... but fat people are more liable to certain illnesses like blood pressure, heart disease ... I don't know" (Naseem).

Others draw on their own experience and trade off the modern and traditional ideas: "Average weight people are healthier than the fat. The fat people have some problems, so do the thin" (Shobha); "Anybody can get illness, any time - fat people, slim people, anybody" (Rani); "You can never really tell who is a really healthy person. Some fat people are healthy, some are ill. Some people who are thin are very healthy. Some people are slim due to the illness, and some are just thin, physically and they are quite active ... You shouldn't be overweight or underweight, just normal weight according to your height" (Tasneem).

Very few of the women were overweight in my estimation. Dalee is the largest, owing to her illness which keeps her virtually house-bound, and she does not think her weight can affect her health - in fact, she is one of the stronger believers in the traditional view that to be overweight is healthier than to be underweight. Similarly, Baji, who is the only other woman to be "overweight", does not see her excess weight as a problem or a cause of her leg pains. Lack of weight, then, is seen by some of the informants to be indicative of ill-health, as the traditional view suggests, but westernization has eroded and is eroding these opinions so that many of the women are no longer sure, or hold both (contradictory) views. Health education may be important here, as the women assimilate modern ideas that weight is harmful to health, but at the same time use their experience to justify adhering to old beliefs. They are caught between two worlds: the world of their tradition and heritage that their husbands and older members of the family wish to retain; and the modern world of their children with which they are becoming increasingly familiar.

The informants are, however, fairly convinced that smoking can only be harmful to health. This probably arises from cultural and social objections to smoking as much as to recent publicity in Britain. Most of the women say that they do not smoke because it is prohibited by their religion, and the others do not smoke because they do not like the smell of it. Six women feel that it can damage the lungs (Rani, Tasneem, Farah, Shobha, Baji and Rajinda); three that it can cause cancer (Sufiya, Dalee and Shobha); and Reena mentions the advertisment concerning the harmfulness of smoking to pregnant women. Only Taresh is not convinced: "Some doctors also smoke and some people who don't smoke have bad health, and some people who smoke still have got health, so I can't really say smoking can cause real illness."

A similar pattern emerges in the informants' attitudes to the issue of exercise. Only Dalee feels that exercise is unimportant, and this is a result of her serious ill-health. Many of the women who stress its importance, however, go on to admit that they cannot or have not got the time to do any exercise: Naseem's back is too painful, Syeda is busy with her children, Tasneem thinks housework is exercise enough, and Farah feels too cold to do any. Rajinda is the only one to go to a regular class to exercise; the others do it at home, including Rani, who feels her prayer is sufficient exercise.

The issues covered in this section show the variable effect that westernization has had on the informants. Most migrated in adulthood, and so have been exposed to both traditional and modern beliefs. Traditional ideas are still held by some about food, remedies, temperature and weight, but others have adopted, almost totally, western views. Some of these and others seem to be able to hold both sets of views, despite their often being contradictory, saying at one stage that they do not believe in traditional views, but then going on to express an opinion that accurately reflects traditional views. The negotiability of the two sets of ideas seems to depend on their personal experience, and both sets can be used to the informant's advantage at different times. In some cases, the informants want to adopt western, "modern" ideas, perhaps to keep up with their children; but in other cases, they want to hold on to traditional practices. It is clear, however, that health education material which conflicts with traditional views will not succeed unless personal experience or the experience of others confirms it, enough to allow the overthrowing of deeply held beliefs.

Living in Britain

Racism

The majority of the informants do not understand English, and some go out of their homes only rarely. Despite this, only five of them say they have never experienced any sort of racial discrimination in Britain. Of these five, two have been in Britain only six weeks (Farah and Farida), one cannot understand English at all (Geeta), and one feels that, "The West Indians are the worst with us - worse than the whites, especially in the hospitals" (Rajinda).

The eight who say they have felt racism directed against them (Naseem, Taresh, Syeda, Rani, Tasneem, Sufiya, Dalee and Shobha) speak mainly of people abusing them in the streets or shops: "Sometimes, in the shops, you feel it, but since I can speak English, if someone is rude to me, I can speak to them, say something back" (Naseem); "Once, when I was going in the street, white youths came and threw eggshells and things at us" (Syeda); "Sometimes the boys pass us and they pass some remarks. We know at heart they are not as good as they should be. The others, may be they have certain grudge about us, but they don't show it so much. They keep it in their hearts, whereas the teenagers, they can't hide it" (Tasneem); "Some of them think we can't say anything at all, can't speak, that we're all the same" (Naseem).

Some of the women have home-helps, and they say that they are treated badly by some of them. The home-helps, they say, although employed by the council, refuse to clean their homes, complaining about smells of curry and making fun of their clothes. Naseem has complained about them, and Dalee feels she has been particularly badly treated: "They don't want to do our work ... They treat us like animals - just speak to us when they have to" (Dalee). Others speak of prejudice that others have told them about. Reena says, "My husband works very hard and he says they still didn't appreciate us and they were prejudiced." Naseem says her husband experiences prejudice at work: "Some people are prejudiced ... Certain people, they don't like dark people superior to them."

The informants live in a part of London which has recently attracted national attention after a group of so-called "vigilante" Asian youths were caught and charged with assaulting plain clothes policemen after the youths had tried to escort younger children to school to protect them from racially-motivated physical and verbal attacks. One of Shobha's children has been involved in the attacks on children: "Some people beat my son at school and broke his finger. After that, I gave a report to the police and the school." She and several of the other women say that their children will have to fight back. Shobha is angry about the attitude of the government too: "Mrs Thatcher says immigrants will swamp the country. The way she talks makes people think we are not good people, but since we came, more jobs are going around. But she keeps on being prejudiced, saying immigrants are spoiling the country, making it dirty. All the things we do for the country and she doesn't take any notice of the work she gets from us." There is a feeling of defiance, also expressed by Taresh: "We are working hard, and we are getting our own money, so we don't care if they treat us well or badly. We know that things happen here and we just have to live with them."

The threat of racist violence (verbal and physical) contributes to the women's loneliness and depression. As Naseem says, "It affects your mind. If you feel depressed that you are not treated as other people are or they look down on you, you will feel mentally ill, won't you? It will depress you that you are not treated as good as you would be in your own country. So if you are not treated well racially, it will affect your health in some way. It will cause you depression, and the depression will cause the illness" (Naseem).

Although the women do not explicitly say that they have experienced racism in the NHS, there is some evidence to suggest that they have. On several occasions, they say that they have been told to be quiet, that they make too much fuss, or that they are pretending to be ill. Naseem says of her treatment in hospital "L": "They couldn't find anything wrong [with the back]. The doctor kept saying I was making too much fuss about nothing. That was Dr Perkins, he said that we people should all be called - that I should be called Mrs Brown because of my colour ... Lots of people say it happens to them as well." Sufiya recalls that whenever she took her baby to the doctor, he would say, "'There is nothing wrong, you are worrying for nothing'" (Sufiya).

Tasneem has also experienced doctors suggesting that she is making too much fuss. She recalls that whenever she was feeling ill, and had undiagnosed pneumonia and tuberculosis, "They thought there was some trouble between me and my husband ... that was making me ill", and doctors went on to say that "Indians" fall ill because they are "all" vegetarians. Shobha was told a similar story: "I ask the doctor if I am allergic or anything, and he just says, 'You better eat a lot of meat.' Nothing else he tells me." It would seem that too many of these informants have experienced this treatment for it to have nothing to do with their colour.

There are indications by the informants that they have been overcharged for some medical treatment because they cannot speak English. At the meeting of women before I started interviewing, several complained that they had been transferred to private treatment without their knowledge and charged heavily for treatment that should have come under the NHS. Similarly, some are made to feel that they should not be receiving the treatment that they are entitled to. Sufiya, for example, said that whenever she went to the hospital with her son or collected his prescriptions or drugs, the medical personnel always mentioned the enormous cost of the treatment for thalassaemia, and said that she was lucky not to be in the sub-continent where the child would probably have died. Dalee and Tasneem also speak of these attitudes . All of these make the informants uncomfortable, and add to their depression. Another consequence is that they are increasingly unwilling to go to their doctors or hospitals because they fear that they will experience more of these unpleasant attitudes, or that they may be treated badly.

Work

None of the women does any paid work outside the home, and only three do any regular home-working. Taresh, Geeta and Shobha do sewing machine work, using their own machines, for a little pocket money. Shobha receives the most money, 60p per dress, and she can make twenty a day; Taresh, on the other hand, works for about five or six hours a day sewing shirts and says that she gets, "very little money"; similarly,

Geeta sews money bags, gets 2p per bag and can only sew about 250 in four or five hours. Geeta says she likes to work, and that she feels, "better when I'm working", but she does complain about the money she receives which is usually about £5 per day. Taresh works hard and feels it can affect her health: "I get pain in the eyes and the muscles in the shoulders because I have to bend for long periods over the machine." Shobha does not think the work will harm her health: "I can stop and start, choose when to do it ... I do it to pass the time", and she can collect £50 in a week.

Of those who stay at home, five say they would like to be able to work (Naseem, Tasneem, Farah, Rajinda and Farida). They cannot, however, because of a lack of English (Farah, Farida, Rajinda); or because of ill-health (Naseem and Tasneem). They would like to work because they feel it would ease the boredom. loneliness and depression they experience at home all day, every day. Some of the women do not want to work: Rani says that her housework is enough for her; Syeda and Sufiya have too much to do looking after their children to work as well; and Reena says that she has never worked and can see no reason to start now. Work, then, is not a major factor in the lives of these informants.

The Environment

The environment of Britain is thought by the informants to affect their health, particularly through the influence of the weather. Five of the informants feel that they are definitely less healthy in Britain than they would be in India or Pakistan, because, "The climate attacks your bones and you get aches and pains in your body more than at home" (Tasneem); because of, "the dampness and coldness in this country. We don't get enough sunshine in this country and we get aches and pains in the whole body" (Baji). Naseem and Tasneem complain especially about the loss of friends and relatives which leads to depression and ill-health. Dalee has been ill only in Britain, and she worries that her husband wants to return to Pakistan, but she cannot because of the treatment she needs.

Rani and Naseem speak particularly of the warmth of Pakistan, and the availability of people to talk to, both things they miss in Britain, and which, they feel, affect their health: "I think most of the illnesses can be helped with the sunshine ... and with the company of other people ... I am sure that some people would be better off if they were not here" (Naseem). "The sunshine in our country makes you perspire a lot and that makes you feel better ... In this country ... you don't have that and you don't feel so good as you do in your own country. In our country, you can get fresh air all the time, but here you have to keep all the doors and windows closed to keep out the cold weather, and this affects your health too" (Rani). Rani goes on to say that Britain has much better housing and a higher standard of living than Pakistan, but that people still get all the diseases, "in spite of all the facilities. So it means that you can get these things everywhere" (Rani).

Four of the informants feel that their health is better through living in Britain. Syeda says so because, "the food we get here is better. They are pure - the butter and the flour is pure, whereas in Pakistan, they sometimes mix things." Rani thinks that most things about Britain are "better" - the medical treatment, the food, the houses and the standard of living. Tasneem and Geeta think it may be better because, "you can get good treatment" (Tasneem), but as indicated above, Tasneem also thinks that the climate in Britain is bad for health. It would seem that in some ways Britain is perceived to be better, but in other ways, it is thought to be injurious to health. It may be that their expectation that Britain would be a healthy place when they were in the sub-continent may be being replaced by their experience of ill-health in Britain. Sufiya, Shobha, Rajinda and Reena think that coming to Britain has had no effect on their health at all, and Farah and Farida have not been here long enough to decide.

A change in the weather or climate, paticularly through a person moving from one country to another is, however, expected to cause some ill-health: "Sometimes the weather suddenly gets cold and you get pains and aches in the body; sometimes it gets suddenly hot, and that can cause illness too" (Shobha). Rani thinks more about a change of climate: "When they go from one place to another they get tummy upsets, diarrhoea because the climate has changed, the water has changed ... Here the weather, the dampness, the lack of sunshine, it gives you aches and pains in the body. In warm climate, like Pakistan, you do sometimes get illness like cholera, sometimes malaria due to the mosquito."

Tasneem is concerned about the apparent, as she sees it, lack of health among Asian women in Britain compared to their white contemporaries: "Our 35 years old will look much older or as old as their 55 year old lady. They look younger than us. May be due to their food and may be they have less worries than us as well." Overall, the informants' lives in Britain are not healthy or happy.

Although a few believe that their lives are better in Britain because of better medical treatment or purer food, the majority miss their friends and relatives and previous homes. Leaving behind relatives and familiar places is difficult, and when compounded by a hostile host population and difficulties with the language, the situation becomes pretty desperate. Although the Asian community in the area they live in is quite large, the common "Asian" descent is not always enough to bring people together: religious, kinship and class ties as well as personality clashes mean that not all the women get on well together, and so loneliness for many is inevitable and pervasive.

The Health Services

NHS Doctors and Drugs

All the informants are registered with an NHS general practitioner, chosen either because of the nearness of the surgery (Syeda, Rani and Dalee), or on the recommendation of friends or relatives (Naseem, Taresh, Tasneem, Sufiya, Farah, Geeta, Shobha, Rajinda, Reena and Farida), or in answer to a doctor who advertised his surgery by leafletting the area (Baji). Five attend a solo practitioner (Naseem, Tasneem, Sufiya, Geeta and Reena), the others attending surgeries with two or more doctors. Four say that they make appointments to see the doctor (Naseem, Taresh, Shobha and Rajinda); Baji says she can either make an appointment or just turn up to see a doctor; and the others just go along and wait.

The majority of informants (eleven) attend only an Asian general practitioner, citing the advantage of being able to discuss their health in their own or some other shared Asian language. Reena suggests that this is better because, "he can speak our language, so he can understand our problem." Two of the women who do see Asian doctors, however, are not happy with them. Baji says that whenever she goes, she always sees a different doctor, but that they all, "just give us the medicine and it's always the same thing." Rani is also dissatisfied: "Sometimes they don't treat you very well, and I want to change. Sometimes the English doctors pay more attention to you than the Indian ones. The English will be better." This is a view shared by the most westernised informants, Naseem and Tasneem, both of whom can speak English well and feel happier consulting British doctors.

Only four of the women emphasise that they would prefer to see a female doctor if they could, particularly for internal examinations (Syeda, Farah, Sufiya and Taresh). The others do not seem to mind seeing a male doctor, so long as they believe he is a good doctor. Sufiya is especially happy to consult her female doctor, and reveals that sympathy and understanding are this doctor's best attributes: "She listens to the patient very well and you feel psychologically better when you talk to her. Half your illness is gone when you talk to her because she is very nice, very friendly, and speaks Punjabi."

Several of the informants indicate that most of their illnesses are connected with their loneliness and depression. Like Sufiya, they prefer doctors who will listen to them, give them enough time to express their worries, and take good care of them. Naseem thinks she has a very good doctor who is always sympathetic and thoughtful, and gives her all the treatment she needs. Similarly, Tasneem is pleased with her GP now, although he failed to diagnose her tuberculosis, because, "the doctor is very careful with me now, after that trouble. Anything I ask for, he gives it." Dalee's doctor also checks on her regularly, and she says, "he is very nice with me, very careful with me" (Dalee). Rajinda knows her doctor well because he was a friend of her husband, and she is confident that he will take good care of her.

Some of the informants, however, are not so pleased with their present or past GPs. Sufiya saw a male doctor before her present one, and she felt that he treated her son badly: "Whenever I used to take the baby, he used to say, 'There is nothing wrong, you are worrying for nothing.'", and on another occasion when she called him out on a holiday, he said, "'you know your child is always ill, why didn't you bring him on

Friday?' That's why I wanted to change doctors - he upset me" (Sufiya). Similarly, Rajinda changed her doctor because she failed to tell her about her daughter's brain damage, used to make her pay for treatment, and once, "when we got some medicine from India, she was angry and she shouted at my husband. That upset him, and we stopped going there" (Rajinda).

Rani, Shobha, Baji and Taresh are also dissatisfied with their GPs. Shobha and Baji complain that, "they are changing the doctors too often", and that, "sometimes they don't try to find out what is wrong" (Shobha). Shobha's doctor's only advice is to eat more meat. Rani complains that her doctor is, "in too much of a hurry", and that, "he treats better those he knows best" - it may be that she attends the same surgery as Rajinda and sees Rajinda getting more time and attention because the doctor knew her husband. Taresh is dissatisfied with her GP because, she says, "Everytime I tell her I am not having proper periods, she says, 'Go for the test, you might be pregnant.' But I am not. Every time she says this, even though I have got the coil ... Six months ago I went to get my coil changed ... I didn't change it during ten years ... She said it will take a few weeks to settle down, so be careful and don't get pregnant" (Taresh).

All of the informants apart from Farida report having seen a GP within the last year. Five saw their doctor some time in the week before the life-story interview: Naseem about pre-menstrual tension; Syeda, "to talk about my general health"; Tasneem because of diarrhoea after a recent trip to Pakistan and Mecca; Sufiya to collect her son's five regular prescriptions; and Dalee called her doctor out to look at her arm which was broken. Four attended a surgery within a month of the interview: Farah to try to relieve her children's toothache; Geeta to collect the iron tablets she takes for anaemia; Baji for pains in her legs; and Rajinda because of a discharge. Rani and Shobha had seen their doctors within the last three months: Rani for a strained back and Shobha for a blood test to see if she was anaemic. Taresh last visited her doctor about six months before, to change her coil; and Reena went a year ago to have the injections she needed to travel to India.

Only five of the women were not taking some drugs when they were interviewed. Seven admitted to taking tablets: Rajinda for insomnia; Dalee water tablets, steroids and blood pressure tablets for her "SLE"; Geeta and Syeda iron tablets for anaemia; Baji water tablets for leg pains; and Reena and Sufiya panadols for headaches. Tasneem said she had a medicine for diarrhoea, and Dalee was also given an ointment for her arm before it was X-rayed and found to be broken.

The informants do not seem to mind in which form the drugs come. A large proportion take tablets and do not seem to mind. There is some preference mentioned for injections, perhaps because some of the anaemic women have had injections that have made them feel better, or because they have become used to having injections either in the sub-continent or when they travel. Rajinda is the only one to express a strong opinion: she feels that she cannot take any medicine or powdered drug because it leaves a nasty taste in the mouth and is difficult to swallow. Some of the informants take vitamin pills - Naseem and Tasneem take "multi-vitamins", and Syeda, Geeta, Shobha and Rajinda take iron tablets, although they do not always take them regularly. Geeta says, for example, that she has been made to take too many iron tablets: "I am taking only one. I feel too hot with three." She is the only one to make explicit the links with traditional ideas about the "heat" of western drugs.

There are some indications that the informants are becoming less willing to go to their doctors. Although they do tend to see their GPs regularly, some very often, they do not always go when they feel unwell. Naseem, Farah, Farida, Dalee and Rajinda say that they will always go to their doctor straight away whenever they feel ill, but the others, most of whom are less happy with their doctors or who say that they have received poor treatment, are not so keen: "I had very bad 'flu ... Many times I meant to go to the doctor, but in the end I dropped the idea, and just took panadols at home and lemon tea" (Taresh); "I always want to go, but in the end, I leave it" (Geeta); "I don't go because he will just give me the same medicine. It's no use going" (Baji); "Sometimes I think I should go, but I just leave it" (Tasneem).

There is, then, a contrast between the women who are happy with their doctors and confident enough to put all their trust in certain practitioners; and those who retain some traditional ideas about health and treatment and have had these confirmed by poor treatment by doctors in Britain. For some, seeing a general practitioner is the first thing to do when they feel unwell, but for others it is a later resort, after the condition has been left, re-assessed and perhaps some self-medication is tried. Again it is personal experience, the degree of sympathy offered by particular doctors and the severity of the complaint which seem crucial to the decision of whether or not to consult a GP.

NHS Hospitals

Seven of the informants report that they have had no experience of hospital treatment for themselves, either in Britain or abroad, and so cannot make any comments (Sufiya, Farah, Shobha, Baji, Reena and Farida). Only two are happy with the treatment they received in British hospitals (Rani and Dalee), and four are very critical (Naseem, Tasneem, Taresh and Rajinda). Five of the informants (Syeda, Geeta, Shobha, Rajinda, Reena and Baji) say that they have only been to hospital for attention to their children and grandchildren.

The two women satisfied with their treatment went to different hospitals. Rani had a gall-stone operation in "L" hospital, and although she can speak no English, says, "They treated me very well ... They brought me an interpreter ... and she explained everything." Dalee has been to several hospitals on many occasions, and she has very few complaints. She goes to "M" hospital regularly for checkups, and is shown to the students: "They do lots of tests on me ... Any exams they have for the students, they send a letter to me. Once they took a piece of my kidney tissue - that was very painful ... I don't mind, I am very happy to go there. It is a rest for me ... It is a change from being at home" (Dalee). Dalee likes hospital "M", but has a complaint about hospital "E" where she was rushed after her second stroke: "There was only one ward for the ladies and gents, and only one toilet for both to use" (Dalee).

Of the six who went to hospital with someone else, only two are unhappy about the treatment they received. Syeda and Shobha went after their children had had accidents; Reena after an accident to her husband; an Baji with a grandchild who had a bad cough. Geeta went with her husband when he cut his hand badly on some glass, and she reports, "still his hand is not straight", and this is of particular importance because he is a carpenter and cannot now do any repairs around the house. Rajinda is the other informant who is unhappy with the treatment her daughter received. Her story is confusing and distressing.

Initially, Rajinda said the death of her daughter occurred because, "she missed her daddy very much and she got a high temperature and chickenpox and complications caused her death." This, however, is the very end of the story. She went on to tell of her attempts to get the truth from "E" hospital and a local clinic, both of which declined to accept responsibility for the child's condition. Rajinda describes what happened: "When she [the daughter] was young, she had the whooping cough vaccine and it damaged her brain. She was not talking until she was two and she could not balance her head at all. Over here, I was taking her to every clinic and they never told us she had any brain damage, but when we went to India, a consultant professor told me her brain was affected due to that injection ... They didn't tell us at all. They sometimes pay damages, but they wouldn't even tell us. She was six months old when we found out about the damage and we stopped going to ... our family doctor because she hadn't told us ... The injection was done here, when she was three months old, and they got a signature from us to say that if anything happened from the injection, they are not responsible ... The people at the clinic said it was not their fault - that she was brain damaged at birth, not by the injection, but the hospital said she was perfect when she was born ... So, instead of doing everything for her, they never even agreed it was their fault" (Rajinda).

At a different time in the interview, Rajinda recalled an incident during childbirth that may or may not be relevant to the above story. She says, "The baby was overdue, so I went into hospital for ten days and I wasn't having any pains at all so they induced the baby - gave me tablets to start the pains, but they stopped again. Next day, they used the tablets again, and the baby arrived" (Rajinda). Rajinda is understandably bitter about the treatment she has received from the local health services.

Tasneem also feels that she was treated badly by the NHS. After the birth of her last child, she says, "I was ... losing weight, lot of weight, and I was getting very tired." She continues that her doctors did not take any notice, but eventually referred her to "E" hospital, where she was treated as an outpatient for a year. At "E" hospital, she says, "They thought there was some trouble between me and my husband ... They asked if I was happy with my husband ... They told my husband to take me out sometimes because I was staying in all the time, and may be this was causing the trouble ... They took X-rays and blood tests ... But they couldn't find any illness at all. After six months, they said there was nothing wrong with me ... Then I started to get temperature, very high temperature, and it went on for a month. One night, I felt a very, very severe pain in my chest and my husband had to call the doctor ... He came and said I've got an attack of pneumonia, so he sent me straight away to "K" hospital [an isolation unit]" (Tasneem).

She continues, "They rang up "E" hospital to find out what was going on before ... They took more X-rays, and said I'd got pleurisy - fluid in the lungs. I must've had this all along, but they didn't find out through the year ... The doctor said I'd been having this trouble for more than a year, when I wasn't putting on any weight and getting out of breath. They should've found out earlier ... They moved me to a special hospital. I stayed there for three months ... They had X-rays of the whole family. At that time they were concerned because they knew it was due to them that the trouble had become worse ... I took medicine for two more years ... They told me it was 'flu and chest trouble, pleurisy, the first stage of TB. I caught TB, you see" (Tasneem).

Naseem's bad experiences of hospital treatment occurred soon after she had arrived in Britain, during and just after the birth of her twin sons who were both breech births. She recalls, "I was not healthy at all during my pregnancy." She describes the delivery: "It was forceps and I was three days in labour pain. It was a bad one and they gave me stitches ... The stitches got septic and they left the afterbirth in ... I was really ill after the deliveries ... I was not experienced at that time at all ... I didn't know what I should do for the hospital people. They were not fair to me at that time" (Naseem).

She continues, talking about hospital "E": "The maternity hospitals are very bad for black people. I was treated badly. They left the afterbirth, and when I came round, I just said, 'Pain, pain', and they ignored me. Then they saw I was all swollen, so they took me to the theatre, and without anaesthetic they did the D&C [dilation and cutterage]. It was so painful. Afterwards they were not helpful either. They gave me some tablets for the milk ... They didn't tell me what they were for. They have given me all the lumps in my breasts ... They aren't very helpful with the Asian ladies - they don't understand their problems. They upset me, and I'm sure they're worse with the other ladies" [she is referring particularly to those women who cannot speak any English] (Naseem).

The final example of poor treatment also occurred in "E" hospital, this time to Taresh. She says that she had an operation on her hand and that, "When I came round, I felt sick ... One nurse was very rude and angry. She said, 'Why are you being sick and saying you feel dizzy and this and that? Nothing is happening to you. You are just pretending that you are being sick. You are making yourself sick.' Then my hand got septic, and I showed it to the nurse and still she didn't agree. The doctor came and saw my hand was swollen and he changed the bandage and I felt better" (Taresh).

The informants were very frightened of going into "E" hospital because of the bad reputation it has among them after the terrible treatment that some of them have received there. By the time of the second interviews, the hospital had been closed and the informants have mixed feelings. Some are glad it has closed and are quite willing to travel to the new hospital, but others are worried that the new hospital is too far away.

Some of the informants are very worried about having hospital treatment because of the stories, like those above, that they have heard. Consequently, they put off going to see doctors about conditions that they think might lead to hospital treatment. It also causes them extra worries, and Reena was terrified about her cataract operation at the time of her interview. The extra worries are cause by a fear of anaesthesia, wondering what will be done to them when they are asleep, and not knowing how they will react to it. Again there is a division, however, between those who have had experience of good treatment and so are confident of NHS treatment, and those who have had very poor treatment and are, therefore, skeptical or openly critical.

Private Medicine

Tasneem's lack of confidence in the NHS is mirrored by her use of private doctors. She has not called them for herself, but usually does so when her children are unwell. She says, "Sometimes my family doctor doesn't give so much medicine for the children, so I, for my own satisfaction, just call the private doctor. He only charges £3 for a visit and then gives a prescription" (Tasneem). Naseem says she would like to see an osteopath about her back, but as yet she has not found anyone who knows the name of a good one. Otherwise, none of the women prefers private practitioners to NHS ones. Only Dalee of the others has seen a homeopathic doctor, and that resulted in real harm to her.

Dalee was in severe pain because of rheumatiod arthritis, and a next-door neighbour suggested that she should see a homeopath she knew. Dalee says, "The first stroke happened because the lady next door told me I should have homeopathic treatment for the pains, this arthritis ... At that time, the doctors had put me on steroids, always I am on steroids. Well, I stopped the steroids to take the homeopathic drug, and then the stroke happened. Now I always take the steroids ... My doctor said that if they could find him [the homeopathic doctor] they will sue him. First of all when I had the stroke, he didn't want to know anything at all. Then later, he said, 'Forget about me, and just go to the hospital'" (Dalee). The first stroke left Dalee paralysed down one side, which makes her virtually house-bound and leaves her unable to do all but the most simple tasks.

CONCLUSION

These, then, are the perceptions and experiences of health, illness and the health services of the informants of Asian descent. Of particular importance to their health are worries, depression, religion, chance, fate germs, food, racism and the quality of health care they receive. Factors such as worries, depression, germs and racism are perceived to have deleterious effects on their health; food and religion to have beneficial effects.

It is clear that these informants suffer from many non-physical health complaints, many of which they feel arise because of their feelings of loneliness and depression, and their worries about things beyond their control. They worry particularly about the futures in store for their children, and things that may be happening to friends and relatives abroad, with whom they can have little contact. The informants have few opportunities to express these worries, and they expect their GPs to have sympathy and to listen to them when they experience any physical complaints, whether these are or are not associated with their mental state.

It is important to bear in mind that many of these informants came originally from quite wealthy or middle-class families, and several have tried to maintain their social position in Britain. Several have found this difficult, facing racism in the employment and housing markets and some hostility from the white population. Some have found that they can only buy homes in "Asian" areas, for example, where they have to mix with different class and religious groups. Kinship, class, religious and personal difficulties mean that not all the women get on with each other, thus adding to the loneliness many of them feel.

The health of the informants, like their lives, is largely determined by factors out of their control. The broad social, economic and political forces that brought them from the sub-continent to settle in Britain, allied to disease-carrying agents such as germs determine their state of health. Their response is limited to trying to eat the right foods to build up the body's defences and to immersing themselves in religious beliefs and practices which give their lives a sense of purpose and give them the strength to cope with the loneliness and worries of everyday life. Their cultural heritage means that some can almost live in two worlds: one of traditional beliefs and practices; the other of modern and western ways and views. Most cannot avoid the modern world even if they want to as their children demand particular foods and possessions, but many do not also want to disown their cultural heritage. Most can, therefore, exercise some choice of actions, within the overall constraints of life in Britain, although it is these constraints which ultimately determine the quality of their lives and health.

PART III
CONCLUSIONS

7 The health of black people: control, context and choice

Introduction

This thesis is concerned with the perceptions and experiences of health, illness and the health care services of two groups of people with different ethnic/cultural origins who are, at present, living in north and east London. So far, three introductory chapters have established the backcloth against which the study is set, a fourth chapter has outlined the methodological principles underlying the conduct of the empirical work, and the fifth and sixth chapters have considered and interpreted the relevant perceptions and experiences of the informants chosen. In the empirical work, the focus throughout has been on the wholeness and uniqueness of individuals, achieved through the analysis of case-studies. The first part of this chapter will discuss the similarities and differences in the perceptions and responses of the two groups of informants. The next part will be concerned with examining further the chosen methodology. The final part will attempt to link the empirical work with the introductory chapters, through the concepts of control, context and choice.

Key Categories Shared by the Informants

There are many similarities between the informants of Afro-Caribbean and Asian descent, despite their quite different cultural heritages and historical origins. The majority of the informants were, for example, born outside the UK, and many share the same opinions on the effects that such things as germs and worries may have on their health. There are also some striking similarities in the informants' views on the effects on health of depression, food, the environment, racism and religion.

As the majority of the informants were born outside Britain, they share the experiences of a childhood abroad, and of migration. Most remember their childhoods as years of health and happiness, although several of the Asian informants mention that they suffered from complaints such as smallpox and typhoid which seem to be accepted as part of life. None of the informants dwell on their childhoods or their teen years, preferring instead to talk about the more pressing concerns of the present and more recent past. The important times in their more distant past seem to be the occasion of marriage, especially for the Asian women, the time of the birth of their first child, especially for the Afro-Caribbean women, and the first job for the Afro-Caribbean men. The experience of migration was also important, although unpleasant, for many.

"Health" is seen by almost all of the informants as a residual state, and particularly as a state of not being ill. Perfect health is thought to be possible in the abstract, but no-one believes that there is actually anyone who has had perfect health. For some, perfect health is the pristine state of the young which is eroded by time, germs and the effects of the environment, particularly the British environment. Although perfect health is not seen to be possible in practice, several of the informants feel that they have had healthy lives, even if they have suffered from quite serious complaints. This contradictory impression arises from the general acceptance of ill-health including some fairly serious occurrences as part of life, as something to be expected and coped with as best a person can.

The feeling of fatalism, of accepting unpleasant events and episodes of ill-health as "natural", as just "part of life" runs through most of the interviews. Religious beliefs play an important role in this regard, and are meshed with fate in controlling the informants' lives. Only three of the informants say that religion is of little importance to them (Farida, Judy and Dalee), and for the others, it largely controls their lives. Faith in a higher being gives the informants a great sense of peace and comfort, and helps them to cope with the stresses and unpleasantnesses which they face in everyday life. In place of questioning why things happen, their faith allows them to accept what happens, and then to get on with life as best they can.

The two groups follow different religions, with the Afro-Caribbean informants being practising Christians and the Asians being Muslims, Hindus or Sikhs, but ultimately they all experience the same pervasive sense of calm and resignation. For some, elements of their lives are determined by their religion, through the proscriptions of foods or actions, or by the organisation of their activities around times of prayers, services or festivals. The emphasis on cleanliness and purity of some of the Asian religions have an impact on the informants' health; as do the prescriptions of the healing churches which some of the Afro-Caribbeans attend. Many religious practices developed out of a concern for good health, such as the law to avoid pork in Islam and Judaism to guard against the risks of food poisoning. Religion can, therefore, have direct, often beneficial, effects on the physical health of the informants, as well as on their mental and emotional states. Perhaps the greatest influence of all, however, is its alleviation of some of the depression, worries and loneliness which affect the informants. Often any alleviation is temporary, but their faith offers much comfort to those who are most affected.

Depression and worries are shared by all the informants. For the Asians, these originate chiefly from their loneliness in Britain and the difficulties of keeping in touch with relatives abroad. The worries and depression of the Afro-Caribbean informants are caused by lack of money, difficulties at work or concerns about relatives in Britain or abroad. Depression and worries are thought by most of the informants to have physical as well as mental manifestations. For example, people can suffer from headaches, pains in the body, insomnia, hypertension and sugar diabetes because of specific or general worries. Worries and depression are also thought by some to lead to mental illnesses such as nervous breakdowns, or to personality changes.

The effects of worries and depression on health are thought to be enormous by all the informants. Many of those of Asian descent say, for example, that these conditions are the most important cause of physical ill-health, and some recognise that many of their feelings of ill-health originate from worries or depression. Many also rely on GPs for minor complaints which they know are caused by worries, and consequently, they expect doctors to be sympathetic and to have time to discuss their depression. The informants of Afro-Caribbean descent also feel that much of their ill-health originates from these conditions, but they use their faith and their desire to work to overcome these feelings and the problems they cause. The physical manifestations, such as high blood pressure and hypertension, remain, however.

Tiredness is seen by both sets of informants as both a sign and cause of ill-health. It is particularly important for the Afro-Caribbean women, most of whom work full-time and also have domestic and child-care responsibilities. For the Asian informants, tiredness is connected with the boredom and loneliness they feel in Britain. They perceive a vicious circle of loneliness causing depression which leads to more worry and thus on to tiredness and back to depression and loneliness. A shock is also thought by many to be an important contributor to ill-health by causing long-term worries as well as initial difficulties. A shock is perceived to have particularly harmful effects on health if it concerns relatives abroad who cannot be easily contacted or visited, and this is especially so when the shock concerns the ill-health or death of someone abroad.

Germs are thought to be a major cause of ill-health by all the informants. They are perceived to be external agents, usually in the air or infecting others, which are likely to attack the body at any time. Germs are typically seen to be passed on from person to person, usually causing illnesses such as 'flu and fever, although they are also held responsible for more serious conditions such as tuberculosis and smallpox. Germs are seen to invade the body according to chance or fate, particularly when a person has been "in the wrong place at the wrong time", and the power of the body's natural resistance is seen to be of crucial importance to some. Only two of the informants give the scientific explanation of the body's defences; the others speak of an unspecified defence system which depends on an individual's strength, the food they eat, their level of cleanliness, and the strength of the invading germ. Some individuals are thought to be more susceptible to germs than others, but the informants are not sure why this should be so, except that it is just "part of life".

The informants are similar in their unwillingness to dwell on the possibility that heredity might affect them. Although most accept that heredity exists and can affect health, none of them wanted to speculate on the complaints that may run in their own families. This may be because of fear or not wanting to know, or because of the stigma attached to having "family illnesses". There is a similar unwillingness to dwell on the causes of complaints, with the informants concentrating more on alleviating the symptoms or effecting a cure. Some, however, have quite well-worked out, non-scientific theories about how the body works which also suggest likely causes and ways to cope. Although most of the informants do invoke specific causes during their stories about particular episodes of ill-health, they tend to feel that fate or God's will are the chief determinants of most of the things that happen to them. When the informants answered questions briefly, they usually expressed the view that they did not know of any specific causes of ill-health. When they told stories, however, most included some causal theory. This finding may be similar to the public and private accounts discovered by Cornwell (1984) and discussed further below.

Cancer is a disease specified by almost all the informants as either incurable, or a condition to be feared. Some of the Afro-Caribbeans have theories as to its origin, but no-one believes it can be cured. The Asians expect that western medicine will eventually find the cause of cancer, and then its cure, but for now it is a condition to be feared, and to be overcome only extremely rarely.

There are very few things that the informants believe can off-set the development of an illness or disease once it has become established. One way of helping to build up the body's defences against ill-health is seen to be to eat the right sorts of food. For some, it is traditional food that is thought to be best; for others it is heavily advertised western food. The Asian informants in particular have been affected by health education literature which criticises their traditional diet. Their children also demand the western dishes which their school friends have. Consequently, some of the Asians are now unsure as to what foods are best for health, with some still cooking traditional dishes for themselves and their husbands, and others eating a completely westernised diet.

The informants of Afro-Caribbean descent also are changing their diets. Only a few still eat a totally traditional diet, and these are convinced that this is best; some others eat a totally western diet; and others eat a mixture of foods. Despite the confusion over the value of particular diets, the informants all believe that what an individual eats can have important implications for their health. Good food is thought to build the body's strength and capacity to defend itself against invading organisms. Specific foods may also act as remedies for certain sorts of illnesses or diseases.

The freshness of food is also thought to be important by many. They remember the freshness of food in the rural communities where some of them used to live or where they have visited, and they relate this to their perception of the healthiness of everyone. The freshness of food thus becomes closely linked to good health. This is compared with the stale and tinned food obtainable in Britain, where most of them also feel ill and can see ill-health in others around them, and so their belief in the value of fresh food is confirmed and strengthened. Several also complain about the way they are obliged to buy frozen food in Britain, because of a lack of alternatives, and that they believe it to be particularly bad for health because of its coldness and lack of goodness.

The concept of balance is often mentioned in the discussions about health and food. Health is conceived of, for example, as a state of balance, and any deviation from this is thought to be a sign of ill-health. A balance of foods, then, can help to maintain health, and if the body becomes off-balance, certain types of foods or remedies can be used to restore it to its "normal" functioning. The concept of balance is particularly important to the informants of Asian descent, especially in their ideas about hot and cold.

The theme of balance is also taken up in the discussions about temperature. All the informants believe that a person's temperature is a good indicator of the presence or absence of ill-health because it is easily measurable. Health is seen to be having a "normal" temperature, and either a low or high temperature is typically seen as the most obvious sign of illness such as fever, 'flu, or more serious complaints such as tuberculosis and typhoid. These observations link with the Asian informants' conceptions of hot and cold which are not shared by the Afro-Caribbean informants.

Balance is also involved in the informants' views on weight where, typically, a stable weight is seen to be beneficial. Again, any sudden loss or gain of weight is indicative of something wrong with the body. For some, the modern view that to be overweight is bad for health seems nonsensical because they believe that if they have always been the same weight, they must be all right. Some of the traditional opinions suggest that to be fat is better than to be slim, perhaps because to be fat was seen in the countries from which they have migrated to be a sign of relative prosperity. The western view, however, suggests the opposite, and several of the informants are now beginning to ascribe to the western rather than the traditional view.

Racism affects all the informants who have been in Britain for longer than a few months. Since the two groups of informants have quite different life-styles, racism tends to affect them in different ways. Those of Afro-Caribbean descent, for example, experience racism chiefly at work, although some say they can feel it everywhere and that it affects them all the time. The informants of Asian descent, however, do not go out to work, and racism affects them in the streets and the shops, through physical and verbal attacks on their children or friends, or through home-helps. If the attacks on both groups are physical, they can clearly cause damage to health through injuries. The majority of attacks are, however, verbal or indirect, and these affect especially the informants' mental and emotional health. Racism adds to the depression that already fills some of their lives, and it contributes to the frustration and loneliness of many. It may also have physical manifestations: Ruby's sugar diabetes, for example.

Racism is a fact of life for the majority of the informants, and many try to ignore it or accept it, and then to get on with their own lives. Again faith has a role to play, particularly in the ways it gives them the strength to believe in equality, and the determination to resist passively attempts to discriminate against them. Religious beliefs give the informants the strength of knowing that they are right and the discriminators wrong, and so they can feel assured in their fight. Racism can thus be partly shrugged off as yet another unpleasant fact of life, and so life can go on. It does, however, contribute enormously to the informants' depression.

All the informants agree that the environment can have important effects on health, although they are not unanimous about the effects of living in London and Britain. None of the Afro-Caribbeans believe that Britain is in any way healthier than the parts of Africa or the West Indies that they know. The Asians, however, are divided between those who think that Britain is better because of its better housing conditions, higher standards of living and purer food; and those who feel it is worse than India or Pakistan because of the climate. All the informants complain about the coldness and dampness of Britain and its consequent effects on health, causing aches and pains, colds and 'flu, and rheumatism. Some feel that they can never be healthy in Britain.

It may be that some of the complaints about life in Britain derive from idealised views of the past in places in which the informants used to live in the Caribbean, Africa and southern Asia. These places are associated with healthiness, warmth, friendliness, fresh food and good company - most of which seem to be missing from Britain. For many, Britain is thus associated with illness, depression, worry, coldness, dampness, stale food, racism and loneliness. These idealised, stereotypical views of places contribute to the circle of depression and/or loneliness, with memories of the past leading to depression, which in turn leads to more thinking about the good times of the past, and leads on to more depression. These findings are similar to those elicited by Cornwell (1984) in respect of the loss of the idealised conception of the community in Bethnal Green. The informants in this study who feel that their lives are better and healthier in Britain are few in number, and they believe this chiefly because they think they can obtain better food and medical treatment in here.

The informants differ substantially in their general attitudes towards health care, but there are a few specific similarities. All were vague about the last time they saw their GP, or the last time they felt ill. This was especially true of the Afro-Caribbeans, who see their GPs relatively rarely. Another similarity lies in the reliance of a large number of informants on long-term medication, despite the apparent abhorrence of drugs on the part of the Afro-Caribbeans. As far as hospital treatment is concerned, there are a similar number of terrible experiences for people in both groups (see chapters five and six for details).

There are, therefore, a number of shared perceptions and experiences among the informants of the two ethnic groups. Some of these relate to their common experiences of migration and being black in Britain; others relate to the modern and/or western ideas they have absorbed beside and/or in place of their traditional cultural beliefs. Despite the quite different cultural and historical origins of the two groups, and their dissimilar lives in Britian, some of their views and beliefs about health and illness are the same. It will be further argued below that the lives of the informants are largely controlled by factors such as the labour market and the policies of the state, and that they are able to exercise some choice over their own actions within societal constraints. When they are able to exercise choice, the perceptions and experiences of the two groups usually differ because are drawing upon their own cultural and personal heritages. Where their lives are determined by outside factors, such as the labour market, racism and other social, economic and political forces, the experiences of the informants are similar. Thus they share many of the experiences of being black in Britain and of having migrated, but have, to different degrees, adopted western beliefs and views to which they have been exposed.

Categories Held Exclusively by Either Group of Informants

Although there are some similarities in the perceptions and experiences of the informants interviewed, it is clear that their very different life-styles, heritages, cultures and attitudes lead to some quite obvious differences. Some categories considered in chapters five and six apply to one group alone, and sometimes the groups have different views on particular categories. The categories exclusive to one or other group include the concepts hot and cold, the use of remedies, the importance of work, the issue of language and the problem of loneliness. The informants have different opinions on the NHS, private medicine, drugs, how the body works, smoking, serious illnesses and exercise.

A major difference between the two groups arises from language. The majority of informants of Asian descent did not speak enough English to be interviewed in that language, and so were interviewed using an interpreter. The issue of language is important, and has some wider implications. Several of the informants of Asian descent feel that they, or others who speak little English, are at a severe disadvantage when they require medical treatment. For those who see non-Asian-language speaking GPs, there is the difficulty of explaining what is wrong, and for those who go into hospital, there are difficulties of not knowing what to expect, and not understanding instructions by medical personnel or what is being done to them. Several believe that, as a consequence of this, they have received very poor and insensitive treatment.

Although there has been some concern about the issue of language, very little has been done in the area in which the informants live. The local authority is supposed to provide interpreters who can help non-English speakers, but in practice they rarely do so, and rely instead on the patients bringing in friends or children who can speak English better than they can, or on medical or ancillary staff who speak the required languages and who happen to be on the wards at the appropriate time. Consequently, many of the informants of Asian descent choose to see GPs who speak Asian languages.

The loneliness that many of the Asian informants feel is partially an outcome of their difficulties with speaking English. The majority of those interviewed spoke very little, if any English, and consequently, they are restricted to making friends with and talking to women in the same position as themselves. Class, kinship and personal differences do not always allow friendships to be made easily, and so the feelings of loneliness, caused principally by their migration away from friends and relatives, are exacerbated by the few available contacts in Britain and the hostility of the local white population.

Loneliness is of outstanding importance to the Asian informants, but has little relevance to those of Afro-Caribbean descent. This is despite their similar experiences of leaving friends and relatives behind when they migrated, and is related to their quite different life-styles. The informants of Afro-Caribbean descent are able to go out to work and to converse and make friends with a wide range of people because they go out more often than the Asian informants, and they share the same basic language with the majority of the population. Those who are religious also go out to pray, and so they meet fellow believers; whereas the Muslim women tend to pray at home alone.

The loneliness of the Asian informants is made worse because their husbands go out to work and their children go to school, thus leaving them alone at home all day. Most of them say they would like the chance to work or to learn English, but the jobs are not there, and the council does not provide any day-school opportunities for them to learn English. The informants of Afro-Caribbean descent say that they would hate to have to stay at home all day, and they fear unemployment greatly. None of the Asian informants can see any chance of alleviating the sense of loneliness they feel, except by planning short trips "home" every couple of years to see their missed relatives.

As indicated above, the informants differ over the importance of work in their lives. Work is of crucial importance in the lives of the Afro-Caribbeans, but has relatively little importance for most of the Asians. Work figures in a large proportion of the interviews with the informants of Afro-Caribbean descent. It was, after all, a major reason for their coming to Britain, and it has remained a crucial concern. All the Afro-Caribbean informants want to be working, and several have great fears of unemployment. Work is important to them as a source of income, as something to pass the time, and as a source of pride and independence.

Work is desired by the Afro-Caribbean informants, and yet it is also acknowledged to be the source of much of their ill-health. The jobs taken by them tend to be low-skilled, poorly paid, often in shifts and in dangerous and/or dirty conditions. Most of them are aware of the effects their work is having on their health or might have in the future, but they all want to keep their jobs. Many say, indeed, that the dangers to health are outweighed by the benefits of working. Also, dangerous conditions are usually accepted as "part of the job", just as other events are "part of life".

Those who are religious also draw strength from their work. Work is used as a yardstick against which an individual can measure her/his health. If a person cannot work, for example, they are considered to be ill. Conversely, to be healthy is to be able to work normally. Hence in their interviews, many of the Afro-Caribbean informants consider that the last time they were ill was when they last stayed off work. The seriousness of a complaint is also measured against the amount of time it forces an individual to take off work.

Paid work is only a minor force in the lives of the informants of Asian descent. For the three who do machine work, work is quite important, but they do it only to earn a little pocket money and they have to work very long hours to make it worth their while. Most of the other informants of Asian descent feel that they have enough housework and child-care responsibilities to keep them occupied, although many find that they have too much free time and get bored and depressed.

The use of home remedies is confined almost exclusively to the informants of Afro-Caribbean descent. The informants of Asian descent prefer to rely on western-trained doctors and drugs, and although some can remember using home remedies or recipes purchased from hakims in their childhoods, none has consulted a hakim in this country. The informants of Afro-Caribbean descent, however, are not so willing to rely on western medicine, and they have a strong heritage of using herbal and home preparations to treat minor and major complaints. Many of these preparations are still used in Britain, and even some of the younger informants who have been born and/or brought up in Britain express an interest in, and use, traditional methods of health care and self-medication.

It is principally the older West Indian women and men who know the most about home remedies, because of their experiences in the West Indies and their position at the head of the family. They can recall many instances of ill-health being cured by preparations passed down the generations, and often these were the only option when modern health-care had to be paid for. Most of the remedies are based on liquids and consist of readily available ingredients such as locally-grown herbs, spices and vegetables. Some preparations are brought from druggists (or health stores in Britain), bottled and with brand-names. Tonics are an important part of traditional health-care, particularly through building the body up to ward off infections or to ensure that the obvious systems - the bowels, digestion, blood circulation and menstrual cycles - keep on working efficiently.

The remedies and tonics are connected to a well-worked out, but non-scientific and sometimes inaccurate, corpus of theories concerning how the body works. The emphasis is on those things that can be monitored or are expected to flow, such as the digestive system, the menstrual cycle and the blood circulation system. These theories are used when ill-health is perceived and some treatment required. In the old days, a liquid such as a herbal tea would be used, but now and in Britain, doctors tend to prescribe drugs in the form of tablets. The majority of the informants of Afro-Caribbean descent, however, express a clear preference for the traditional form of drugs - liquid medicines - and this preference is re-inforced by their theories of how the body works, particularly those which suggest that liquids flow to the point of the sickness or injury, whereas tablets have to dissolve before they can have any effects. A consequence of these beliefs is the reluctance on the part of many of the informants to take the prescribed number, if any, of the pills their doctors recommend. The beliefs also strengthen their skepticism of the abilities of western medicine and drugs. Only personal experience that, for example, pills work, can overcome the traditional, cultural preference for liquids. Ruby, for example, declares that she only believes in liquid medicines, but she also takes a pill to control her asthma and she admits that it is the only thing that has ever helped her.

The informants of Asian descent do not seem to have any such well-worked out theories about how the body works. They tend to prefer to rely on the "experts", the medical professionals who are trained in modern techniques. Also, they do not express a strong preference for any particular type of drug, although Rajinda will not take medicine, and some of them do not take the prescribed number of tablets because of the thought that western drugs are "hot". Some say that they prefer to have injections where possible, perhaps because these are quicker and the informants are used to them, having to have various "shots" when they travel to the Far or Middle East.

The concepts of "hot" and "cold" are of great importance only to the informants of Asian descent. To those of Afro-Caribbean descent, these concepts refer only to the feeling of a fever or a high temperature, when a person feels alternately hot and cold. For the Asians, however, hot and cold pervade many of their perceptions of health and illness, their notions of treating ill-health, and the importance of food. The theme of balance is crucial here, with a perception by the informants of a need to balance the opposing forces of hot and cold in order to maintain health. Any deviation from this "normal" state of balance is thought to signal the presence of ill-health.

Balancing the humours of the body is a traditional theory, and it has been developed in southern Asia to cover many aspects of health and health-care (see Davis and Aslam, 1980; Eagle, 1980; Aslam et al, 1981). If the body somehow becomes imbalanced, foods and drinks of the correct temperature can be taken to restore the balance. For example, a high temperature can be off-set by drinking cold fruit juice. Certain foods in excess are thought to be able to cause ill-health: too much chicken and dried fruit, for example, can raise the blood pressure because they are hot foods. As indicated above, western drugs must not be taken in large quantities because they are hot, and so some of the informants do not take all their prescribed tablets.

Some of the informants are becoming skeptical of some of these traditional theories because they run counter to western ideas. Nevertheless, the theories do persist, and some of the informants can see that there are practical reasons for their development, and, in some cases, they accord with western theories. Tea and coffee, for example, are considered to be "hot", to cause damage to the stomach lining and to result in insomnia - all theories with rough equivalents in scientific research.

As indicated above, there is a major difference between the two groups in their attitudes towards the NHS and western medicine in general: the Afro-Caribbeans being skeptical of its benefits, and the Asians being confident in it. The reasons for this difference lie chiefly in the range of options open to the informant. Those of Afro-Caribbean descent have in their families a range of remedies and traditional ideas which can be used to their benefit, depending on the context of the episode of ill-health, or they can choose to see a GP or visit a hospital. Those of Asian descent, however, have dropped many alternative methods of health-care and choose to rely almost totally on their GPs and local hospitals.

The informants of Afro-Caribbean descent may have retained some traditional methods of health-care as a reaction to the poor or unsatisfactory treatment they have received. They have also retained the option of trying out private practitioners when they feel they need them, especially in so far as the NHS does not fulfil their expectations. The informants of Asian descent have also received poor and insensitive treatment, but as they have no alternative methods of health-care, they tend to persevere with their GPs or to change their doctors on the recommendation of friends or relatives. Only two of them have consulted private doctors, but the disastrous effects of the homeopath's treatment of Dalee has convinced most of them that the NHS is best.

The reaction of the two groups to the use of private medicine is worth considering further. The Afro-Caribbeans are all in the "lower" social classes, having typically manual, "working class" jobs and low incomes, whereas the Asians are a mixed group, but with the majority fitting more into the "middle" class because of their higher incomes and husbands' non-manual occupations. It is not, however, the better off Asians who choose to use private doctors, but the less well off Afro-Caribbeans. The willingness of the Afro-Caribbean informants to consult private doctors is linked, according to them, to what the older informants were used to in the West Indies. Then, they say, they had to pay for medical treatment, and so that is what they are used to. They also feel that they are likely to be treated better by someone whom they are paying directly. The younger Afro-Caribbean informants emphasise their belief that "money talks", based perhaps in their parents' experience of state and private treatment.

The Asian informants, however, with the exception of Rani and Tasneem, do not believe that payment will get them better treatment, and Tasneem only sends for a private doctor to look after her children. The reluctance of the Asians to use private medicine for themselves may be linked with their experiences of having to pay for treatment for their relatives when they come from abroad, or it may be that they do not feel that they suffer from anything serious enough to merit paying for treatment. For conditions perceived to be serious, some of them will use private specialists. When Rani became ill with rheumatoid arthritis, for example, she went to a private homeopath; and Naseem, having become almost housebound because of her slipped disc, has decided to approach a private osteopath. It may also be that the limited mobility of the Asian women mitigates against their seeing private doctors, whereas the Afro-Caribbean informants travel more frequently and freely and can thus more easily locate surgeries.

There is a difference in the attitudes of the two groups to ill-health. Those of Afro-Caribbean descent emphasise the need to carry on and bear ill-health as part of life, or to just ignore common complaints which are unpleasant but which do not interfere with the ability to work. Consequently, the informants of Afro-Caribbean descent sometimes found it hard to talk about ill-health because they tend to shrug it off. Without the need to be ready for work, those of Asian descent do not have this to force them to ignore complaints, and because they have time to worry about how they feel, ill-health and discomfort become of great importance to them. Ill-health is related, not to the ability to work, but to tiredness, pain in the body and depression. While the Afro-Caribbean informants seem to have the strength to <u>bear</u> ill-health, the Asian informants seem to wilt under the strain.

This difference in attitude and response to perceptions of ill-health is exhibited in the higher rates of ill-health reported by the Asian informants in their interviews and to their GPs. It is also reflected in the higher rates of psychological complaints mentioned by the Asian informants, and in their concern with mental as much as physical ill-health. For the informants of Afro-Caribbean descent, physical complaints seem to matter much more, although worries and depression are also regarded as a substantial cause of ill-health. These findings have been confirmed by others (see Coupland, forthcoming). There is also a difference in the attitude of the informants towards serious illnesses. Those of Afro-Caribbean descent largely answered negatively, even though some of them had had operations such as hysterectomies, whereas the Asian informants were more willing to specify conditions such as anaemia and severe headaches as serious conditions.

The differences in the perceptions of ill-health may be related to the class of the informants. As indicated above, the Asian group has more "middle" than "working" class members, and they exhibit the higher rates of reported minor ill-health found among members of the white "middle" class (Townsend and Davidson, 1982). The Afro-Caribbean informants seem to suffer from more ill-health, but report it less frequently and willingly, as do the white "working" class (Townsend and Davidson, 1982).

The differences in the perceptions and experiences of the two groups are also closely related to their historical and cultural backgrounds. Although most share the experiences of a life abroad and migration to Britain, they come from quite different places with vastly different cultures, histories, religions and traditions. In some cases, the informants' experiences are similar because of their shared situation of being black in Britain, but when they have the chance to exercise choice, their perceptions and opinions can be quite different and depend upon their cultural inheritance and level of westernisation. In general terms, the informants of Afro-Caribbean have largely accepted western ideas, but have chosen also to maintain some traditional beliefs, whereas the Asian informants are still adopting western ideas as they hear about them but are much more convinced of the efficacy of "progress" and western ways. The reasons for this may lie in the fact that the informants of Afro-Caribbean descent have usually been in Britain longer than the others, and so they have reacted to the hostility of the British and the insensitivity of the health services by retaining and developing traditional ideas and remedies. The reasons for the retention or rejection of traditional beliefs is pursued further below, after an evaluation of the methodology of the study, to which we now turn.

An Evaluation of the Methodology

As indicated in chapter four, the methodology for this project is derived from the ethnographic tradition in anthropology and interpretative sociology. Positivism and structural-functionalism have little to offer the study theoretically or methodologically because the focus here is on the individual and her/his interpretations and experiences of the world. The emphasis throughout has been on an attempt to understand the meanings of health and illness to the informants and the ways in which they make sense of their lives, particularly when their health is threatened. Social facts are not viewed as things, but as the practical outcome of the routine practices and experiences of people in their everyday lives. The study is focused on individuals as case-studies, so that their attitudes towards health and illness can be considered within the overall context of their lives.

The only contribution that structural-functionalism has for this project lies in Parsons' conception of the importance of the relationship between work and health (Parsons, 1951). The lives of the informants who work are largely controlled by the work that they do, and they tend to perceive their health in terms of their ability to work. Ill-health, or the adoption of the sick role, then, is justified or legitimated only when it prevents an individual from fulfilling her/his employment obligations. Many of the informants consider that they are ill when they are forced to take time off work. They are not, however, willing to submit completely to the designs of the medical profession as Parsons postulated, preferring instead to use home remedies or rest in order to recover; and they are also clearly aware that the consultation between the doctor and themselves is not equal or reciprocal.

The ability of the Afro-Caribbean informants to drop their social responsibilities when they are ill also varies according to sex. Parsons postulates that the sick individual becomes labelled "deviant" and is then relieved of her/his social obligations, and although this is largely true for the Afro-Caribbean men, it is not so for the women. The Afro-Caribbean women can stay off work if they are unwell as can the men, but unless the episode of ill-health is incapacitating, the women are still obliged to carry out their domestic and childcare duties.

The variability of meanings of health and illness is due to a large degree on the negotiability of social order. An informant may, therefore, negotiate with others to convince them that she/he is ill and deserves attention. The negotiability of the meaning of ill-health depends on the context of each event. It is clear, for example, that not all episodes of feeling unwell become defined as "illness" or "disease". Hence the young Afro-Caribbean men shrug off minor complaints so that they can go to work, whereas in similar straits one of the lonely Asian informants may consider herself to be ill. In another case, Naseem's back injury has to be ignored by her because she is obliged to make arrangements for visitors. It may be that these differences in perception are related to whether or not the informant feels she/he is responsible for a particular condition (see also Cornwell, 1984). It may be, for example, that Carlton will ignore a cold that he feels he has brought on himself, but complain about one that has struck "out of the blue". Personal blame does not, however, seem to fit in all cases, and there are differences between the two groups. The social context within which the illness has occurred seems to be of immense importance. The Asian women, largely because of their loneliness and boredom, tend to complain of many more illnesses than the Afro-Caribbeans, who have their jobs to cope with as well as their family responsibilities. It may also be the case that class is involved here, with the Asian women complaining of more ill-health because they are more "middle" class.

Power is important in the negotiability of meanings. Doctors, for example, hold power in any consultation with a patient, and often it is they who ultimately decide who is legitimately entitled to the label "ill". Doctors may, for example, contend that a person is not ill according to their criteria, and so social sanction to stay off work or to drop social obligations may be withheld from someone who is clinically "ill". A clear example of this is the case of Tasneem who had TB, but whom doctors diagnosed as having only marital problems. Millie's story is another example of power being used by doctors to deny that she was ill. Her repeated visits to hospital were ignored by doctors who felt that she was overreacting. Similarly, several of the Asian informants mention occasions when doctors have told them they are perfectly all right, but are pretending to be ill. It may be that the power exerted by doctors over black and women patients is a manifestation of race, class and sex relations.

Phenomenology allows that every individual has a unique state of knowledge, based on previous experiences and inherited ideas. These stocks of knowledge can be altered by interactions, through negotiation. Stocks of knowledge also seem to be able to contain contradictory ideas, some of which may be imposed by the dominant meaning systems. The informants in this study have stocks of knowledge which contain theories and experiences from southern Asia, Africa and the Caribbean, some of which have been retained, some discarded, and some maintained alongside contradictory western theories.

The informants' stocks of knowledge allow them to cope with episodes of ill-health. Many of the Afro-Caribbean informants make use of their range of home remedies and self-medication techniques, and assert their preference for liquid medicines. The Asian informants, however, rely more on western medicine, although they still make use of traditional theories about hot and cold which do not fit western ideas. The informants' stocks of knowledge thus allow them to choose between recipes for action.

Schutz's theories, particularly those contained in The Phenomenology of the Social World, are of relevance to this project. Schutz maintained that each individual's stream of consciousness had no intrinsic meaning, but that once an experience had passed, it would be lifted out of the stream of consciousness to become a distinct entity endowed with meaning. This suggests the value of using in-depth interviews which give rise to story telling: only an experience which has passed and been evaluated can be understood and related. Thus the informants were able to talk easily about recent episodes of ill-health such as operations or 'flu, but found it difficult to specify how they felt at the time of the interview.

Schutz developed the idea about individuals' stocks of knowledge to suggest that they provided individuals with "recipes" for action. A perception of ill-health, for example, would then be subject to a set of questions designed to discover whether the symptoms fit a recognised pattern of a specific illness, whether they are unusual, or whether they are just part of life and need to be ignored. Whichever the outcome of the initial investigation, a recipe for action will be available. If the symptoms fit a known illness, for example, self-medication may be tried or a GP consulted. If the condition is perceived to be unimportant, presumably life will carry on as usual.

The form and pattern of these recipes for action will depend for the informants in this study on the individual's stock of knowledge, which will include family and cultural remedies, traditional theories, and a varying degree of westernisation. The degree of westernisation and the presence of traditional theories will allow the informants to have quite different recipes from, for example, an individual with several generations in Britain and a member of the middle class. Some of the theories or recipes will be indexical: they will convey a large amount of information and meanings through a single concept. One such is the "heat" mentioned by some of the Asian informants. A perception of something as "hot" conceals a mass of traditional ideas which need not be explained to those conversant with them, but which seem incomprehensible to the ignorant.

The indexicality of accounts is also a focus for the school of ethnomethodology, as is the equality of concepts. Ethnomethodologists maintain that lay perceptions and opinions are as valid as professional ideologies, although they may be quite different. Lay perceptions of health and ill-health form the bulk of the empirical work in this project, and of particular interest is the way in which they have been affected by western professional medical ideologies. Many of the informants of Asian descent have, for example, accepted professional medical definitions of illness and disease, but at the same time, have retained many of their traditional perceptions. Their lay perceptions, then, are often a mixture of the two distinct ideologies, some of which are contradictory. They accept on the one hand that an illness may be caused by a virus because that is what their doctor has told them, but at the same time, they may still be of the opinion that it was caused by too much "hot food". If asked what they thought the cause of the condition was, they are likely to invoke the doctor's explanation: a virus. If, however, they are telling a story about the experience of the illness, they may well specify the traditional explanation: too much hot food. This may be another example of the differences between public and private accounts found by Cornwell (1984), or it may be that it is the context of the discussion that is crucial.

The ability to manipulate two different belief systems is considered in Cicourel's work on basic and surface rules (Cicourel, 1964). Basic rules are postulated to be deep structures which enable individuals to make appropriate and even innovative responses to changing, unexpected situations. Surface rules, on the other hand, are shallow structures which constitute the tried and tested recipes used in everyday life. Some of the informants of Afro-Caribbean descent have a wide range of tried and tested remedies which they use if anyone in the family feels unwell and if the illness fits an accepted pattern of symptoms. If the illness is unusual or is not affected by self-medication, then medical professionals may be consulted. The informants of Asian descent tend, on the whole, to think of consulting GPs at an early stage in the perception of ill-health, and again this is especially so if the condition is abnormal. It would appear, then, that in the field of health and illness, western medicine is taking over the role of individuals' basic rules. The power of the medical ideology lies in its gradual taking over of people's lives (Illich, 1976), and in its determination that doctors will be the only ones with knowledge of safe health-care.

Western medical ideology has not, however, completely taken over the lives of these informants. Their own experiences of the success of other, traditional methods of health-care, combined with their own beliefs and the sometimes insensitive and poor treatment they have received in the hands of western medicine, has meant that some traditional practices and theories have been retained. Hence some of the informants of Afro-Caribbean descent still use herbal remedies which they believe to be effective, and some have theories about how the body works which are quite distinct from scientific theories and which provide a guide to understanding and responding to ill-health. Similarly, the informants of Asian descent have retained theories about the concepts hot and cold, and some have a traditional attitude towards weight.

The negotiability of the traditional and western medical theories can be seen throughout the interviews. If doctors suggest causes of ill-health which do not fit the informants' beliefs, the doctors' prescriptions and/or advice are often ignored or only partially adhered to. Thus Delores refused to accept her doctor's insistence that the menopause was the cause of her period problems; and Tasneem rejected the doctor's idea that her exhaustion and chest pains were caused by problems with her marriage. Similarly, Geeta refused to take her full quota of pills for anaemia because she believed western drugs are "hot"; and Ivy and Delores do not take as many pills as they should because they do not like taking pills and do not always feel that they need them.

Phenomenology and ethnomethodology have been forceful in criticising positivism and providing alternative theories, but they have, however, been weak in defining and providing a method for empirical work.

Weber suggested the method of "verstehen", to empathise totally with the subject, but this is more an ideal method than a practical one since it calls on the researcher to take on the views and opinions of the informant, and to see the world as if they were looking through the subject's eyes. A researcher may be able to empathise with an informant to a degree, but it is not possible to see the world "as if" one is another person. Empathy with the informant is, however, an important aspect of a qualitative methodology, particularly when interviewing in order to attain the informant's trust. It was of crucial importance in this project.

Schutz developed some of Weber's ideas in an attempt to provide a workable method for sociological phenomenology. Schutz suggested that researchers should study the meanings and perceptions of the subjects through the concepts of ideal types, against which reality could be compared, and scientific or second order constructs which are derived from individual's perceptions. The researcher is obliged to interpret the subject's actions and perceptions by putting her/himself in the place of the other and imagining selecting the same recipes for action. In this way, an individual's actions and perceptions become more comprehensible. This is the method employed in semi-structured interviewing, when the meanings of phenomena are the focus of attention and the interviewer is able to follow up and probe to uncover minor details in order to aid her/his understanding.

The interpretation of the data generated by the interviews follows the pattern established in grounded theory by Glaser and Strauss (1967). Here, the data are used to generate categories such as the definition of ill-health, or germs as a cause of ill-health, against which the data can be compared. As the data are collected, categories are assessed to ensure that they are representative of the data, and if they are not, reasons are established and/or the categories altered. During the collection of data, several categories were dropped because they did not fully fit the data, or else new categories emerged because the data were there to support them. The category of pregnancy, for example, was initially part of adult health for the female informants, but it soon became clear that it had more to do with teenage than adulthood, and was not of crucial importance to many of the women as a health "problem".

The method for generating the data depends on the theory being developed and on logistical questions. Qualitative data are generally obtained through participant observation or in-depth interviewing, or a combination of the two. In this project, in-depth interviewing was the chosen method because the aim of the study is to understand the informants' perceptions and experiences of health and illness, related in their own words, and because participant observation was impossible owing to the difficulties of a white researcher penetrating effectively a black social network. The focus was also on past experiences which had been reflected upon, and which could be relatively easily discussed in in-depth interviews.

Ethnography stresses the influence that the researcher can have on the data and informants. The emphasis is on being faithful to the phenomena under study, and for the researcher to examine all her biases and effects during the interviews. The aim is for the interviewer to take on a "child-like" role, to be a learner, gaining detailed information from the subjects using the skills of prompting and encouragement during the interviews, but also to be critically aware of the content of the dialogue. The data are gathered through in-depth interview which allow the subject to direct the line of questioning, and allow the researcher to alter the presentation and order of questions depending on the subject's responses. The interviews thus progress somewhat like normal conversation, with the emphasis on dialogue rather than on a question and answer session. Although it is acknowledged that the researcher can direct the interview, the aim is to ensure that the informant has the power to choose what and how much to say.

The value of using semi-structured questions rather than a structured social survey instrument comes through clearly in this project. Initial questions, for example, concerning opinions of GPs and hospital treatment were generally answered favourably, but after probing, stories about particular experiences revealed strong complaints and a high level of dissatisfaction. There was a similar unwillingness on the part of the informants to specify causes of episodes of ill-health, but in their stories about other episodes, theories about causes emerged. These are examples of the differences between immediate, surface answers and considered, experientially-based responses, and they have been found elsewhere (Cornwell, 1984).

The use of key informants proved to be an important factor in the project. The child-adult relationship between myself and both Naseem and Delores meant that I could learn about the groups and have access to other people through them. It also meant that I could be trusted by the informants, because they always knew I had been seen by their friends or relatives, and so confidential material was open to me. In many cases, the informants had stories they wanted me and others to know about, and they were prepared to use me as a mediator.

The major advantage of using snowball sampling was that stories could be checked and validated by comparison with others. It also allowed the assessment of the importance of family relations in health and illness, and the degree of retention of traditional views within family or friend groups. Delores's family, for example, shared many ideas on the causes of cancer, the value of certain remedies and the importance of work, but it is only Delores who acts as the point of referral for family health worries. Her children have adopted some of her recipes for action, but she is still referred to in most cases. Joe and Jean's family are similar, and it seems likely that many of the remedies remembered and used by the older generations will be lost when they die. Some of the younger informants use the simpler remedies, but they have largely absorbed scientific theories about the way the body works, and most do not have the detailed knowledge of traditional patterns of health-care that their parents do.

The focus throughout in the empirical work was on the wholeness and uniqueness of individuals through case-studies. The research was carried out as a process in the ethnographic tradition, and the emphasis has been on empathising with the informants while at the same time being aware of the effects I as the researcher may have had. Central to the project is the understanding of the meanings and experiences of health, ill-health and health-care of the informants, and especially the negotiability of these meanings according to the context of everyday events, the effects of social forces and relations, and each individual's personal and cultural inheritance.

The Health of Black People : Control, Context and Choice

Three concepts have emerged repeatedly throughout the introductory chapters, in the empirical work, and in the discussion above. These are control, context and choice. The health of black people in Britain depends on a combination of all three. Many black people are forced to work in often dangerous and dirty conditions, to live in unhealthy environments and housing conditions and to suffer the hostility of the white population and institutions. These factors act as controls on their health, things they cannot affect by their own actions, but which affect their lives. Their lives are not, however, entirely controlled. The context of an episode of ill-health, for example, largely determines whether or not it will be perceived as an illness or disease, and this, in turn, determines whether or not action will be taken to alleviate the symptoms of effect a cure. The personal and cultural inheritances of the informants provide recipes for action and traditional theories that can be used if and when they are required, in place of or alongside western theories and methods. These form the choices the informants can make to affect their health.

The concepts control, context and choice are not mutually exclusive, and the definitions reported below are not suggested to be definitive. There are, in fact, some distinct overlaps. Racism, for example, is cited as a control factor in the informants' lives, but as well as acting as a constraint on their lives, it also forms part of the context within which they live. Similarly, religion is cited below as a choice of the informants, but it also acts as a control over parts of their lives, particularly their attitudes and behaviour. Work can also be seen to transcend the concepts: it is a control because of the limited availability of jobs for the informants; it is a choice because they can choose (in theory) whether or not to take a job; and the context of their work and working conditions are crucial to the understanding of the origins of many of their attitudes towards health and illness, and of specific health problems, mental and physical.

The sections below outline separately the effects of control, context and choice on the informants' lives and health in order that the concepts can be more easily defined and explained; it must be emphasised that these concepts are not mutually exclusive but that they are complex and often intricately inter-related.

Control

A major control in the lives of these informants is the history of immigration and race relations in Britain. It affected the two groups initially in different ways: those of Afro-Caribbean descent were drawn to Britain in search of work or to join family members who had already arrived to find jobs; whereas the women of Asian descent largely arrived later to join husbands or families, many of whom had originally intended to return to southern Asia but who were obliged to stay by immigration legislation which meant that they had to register as British citizens or face future deportation (see chapter one). Many of the informants of Afro-Caribbean descent, therefore, migrated originally by choice; whereas many of the informants of Asian descent did not - some, indeed, were forced out of Kenya.

As indicated in chapters five and six, none of the informants remember migration as a happy or pleasant period, and some have since found little happiness here. The reservoir of negative images about black people originating from the imperial period, combined with anti-black immigration and nationality legislation, led to the development of a hostile attitude on the part of many white Britons and British institutions. From time to time, these attitudes have been fed by political speeches by Enoch Powell, Margaret Thatcher and Harvey Proctor, for example, or media coverage, such as after the reporting of "mugging" as a "black" crime (see chapter one; Hall, 1978; Hall et al, 1978; CCCS, 1982).

An insidious form of control which acts on the informants is racism. This is the theory which encourages or allows the unequal treatment of some people on the basis that they are inferior or different. Because of institutional and personal racism, the informants are constrained in their choice of jobs, areas of residence, housing and so on because of the colour of their skin, (see chapter one, Smith, 1977; Sivanandan, 1982; Brown, 1984). Many of the informants cite clear cases of racial discrimination that they have experienced. This is particularly so for those of Afro-Caribbean descent because they are more active in the labour market and they have generally been in Britain longer. Several of the informants of Asian descent, however, also specify incidents of verbal or physical racial harrassment.

There is some evidence in chapters five and six that racism also affects the informants in the health services, through poor and insensitive treatment, or in the attitudes of medical personnel. As outlined in chapter one, racism affects the lives and health of black people through hostile attitudes, work, housing, education, health and social services and in attitudes towards family composition. For the informants in this study, all of these are relevant.

Work is a crucial variable in the lives of the informants of Afro-Caribbean descent because their lives revolve around its demands and their health is controlled by the type and conditions of work. As shown in chapter one (and Smith, 1977; Runnymede Trust, 1980; Brown, 1984), people of Afro-Caribbean descent tend to be concentrated in particular sectors of the work force and at specific levels, and this is true of the informants. Many of the informants work in dirty or dangerous conditions - the old people's home, a toolmaker's workshop, a British Rail shed, a chemical factory, for example - and these have severe effects on their health, from minor injuries to the groin and back (Leroy and Ivy), to possible asbestos poisoning and exposure to carcinogenic chemicals (Joe and Louise). The informants are largely low paid, and few are in skilled jobs or at supervisory levels. Many work shifts, including those at the old people's home who also have a supervisor whom they consider racist to contend with. Several report discrimination at work, or when they applied for jobs or sought promotion. Although the majority enjoy their work, racism and the jobs they have act as important controls on their health, and have very few beneficial effects.

The informants of Asian descent are also affected by work, although to a lesser degree. Many would like employment, but because of the lack of opportunities and a lack of English teaching, few are able to get it. Those who do work are clearly open to exploitation: as homeworkers, they are ununionised, have to provide their own machines, are not insured, have no security and they can be paid at the rates the employer sets because they have no power to improve their pay or their conditions.

Black people also tend to be concentrated in certain areas of the inner cities (see chapter one, Lee, 1977; Brown, 1984). In part this is a result of the job opportunities open to them; but it is also the result of the availability of housing and some element of choice. The informants in this study are members of distinct communities in two different parts of London. Those of Afro-Caribbean descent are to be found in north London, chiefly on the older, more run down, council estates dating from before WW2; whereas those of Asian descent are in east London, in an area of relatively cheap Victorian terraced houses. Two of the Afro-Caribbean informants (Judy and Emily) complain about their housing conditions, but on the whole, the informants are happy with their flats or houses and do not want to move away from the areas they know well and where their friends live.

The environment of Britain is seen to be a controller of health by many of the informants. The inner-city areas in which they live are polluted and compare unfavourably with the parts of the world from where they or their parents migrated. Many of the instances of ill-health suffered by the informants are blamed on conditions in Britain, particularly the cold and damp weather. A few of the Asian informants believe that Britain is a healthier place than either India or Pakistan, but the others are largely convinced that they cannot expect good health in Britain.

The informants who have themselves or whose children have been educated in Britain are not altogether pleased with it. Some of those of Asian descent complain that their daughters have to go to co-educational schools while they would prefer them to attend all girls' schools. Many also mention that the schools in the area do not make provision for mother-tongue learning, so that this has to be done, where possible, within the community, and some also say that they think their children are not given sufficient help with English. The informants of Afro-Caribbean descent educated here feel that their schools did little to help them, and most feel that they should have done better and achieved more because they have not gained the qualifications they needed to do the jobs they really wanted to do.

The stereotypical concept of black families can act as a constraint on the lives of the informants. The professionals (medical and others) with whom the informants come into contact often have unfavourable stereotypes of black people and their family patterns (see chapter one; Donovan, forthcoming), and these may affect the ways in which they are treated. Afro-Caribbean families tend to be seen to be matriarchal in structure and to be the product of a "weak" culture, a poor imitation of the mother country, England (see Lawrence, 1982). Conversely, Asian families are stereotypically seen to be "strong" and patriarchal, with extended families built around the oldest man. Asian women are usually thought of only as submissive wives, totally dependant on their husbands (see Khan, cited by Parmar, 1982; Allen, 1982).

Stereotypical views of black family life have emerged in the research reviewed in chapter three. Hence the "weak", "uncaring" one-parent Afro-Caribbean family derived from the Moynihan Report (Rainwater and Yancey, 1967), has been used to "explain" the so-called "criminality" of black youth (Pryce, 1979; Lawrence, 1982a), and for high child accident rates (Patterson, 1964). These stereotypical impressions have also been used by professionals when they have been treating these informants. Millie, for example, believes that she was forced to have a contraceptive coil because she is a single black mother. Earl, Carlton, Paul, Danny and Leroy also mention that they have had their cars stopped on numerous occasions by the police who have searched them for drugs or stolen property. Ruby feels that her son was sent to prison owing to the courts not believing her and her son's stories because they are black.

The stereotypical view of the Asian family sees it to be typically extended and dominated by men. It is criticised particularly because it is thought to be rigid and resistant to change (see chapter one). As far as these informants are concerned, these stereotypes are incorrect, as the majority of them live in nuclear family units and their husbands have very little power in the domestic sphere. Rani's husband was present during the interviews, but his presence did not make Rani submissive - on the contrary, when he mentioned something she did not want to hear, she swiftly silenced him and took over the conversation. Similarly, Shobha has fought to keep her nuclear family against the wishes of her husband who wanted to have his parents to live with them.

The informants have, however, been affected by these stereotypes. Tasneem, for example, was told that her chest pains were probably anxiety because of problems in her marriage (the stereotypical view being that arranged marriages cannot be happy), and treatment was delayed for some time before it was discovered that she actually had TB. The assumption that Asian women always want to see female doctors is also not borne out by this research. On the whole, the women wanted good doctors, and most preferred a doctor who could speak an Asian language, but only four said specifically that they wanted to see female doctors. In many cases, the women felt that they had been negleted by the hospital staff when they were ill, and often comments were made to them suggesting that Asians always make too much fuss and that they exaggerate their pain.

The exposure of these stereotypes as untrue among these informants at least is one of the most important findings of this research. These stereotypical views are pervasive and strong, and carry with them many dangerous implications. In the medical sphere, for example, they can cause a person's ill-health to be ignored or misdiagnosed because of the expectations of a doctor or nurse about "Asians", "Afro-Caribbeans" or "immigrants". These stereotypes are not always consciously formed and they can be held by people who believe they are doing their best, but they are, nevertheless, an important and insidious form of racism which needs to be combatted if it is not to continue to have severe effects on black people's lives and health.

Sometimes the demands of family members or social obligations can also act as a control in the informants' lives and can affect their health. Naseem, for example, was unable to rest the slipped disc in her back because she had to make arrangements for visitors and to continue to look after her family, and consequently, she is now in constant pain because of the injury. The demands of domestic duties and employment sometimes leave the women of Afro-Caribbean descent completely exhausted, and this is especially severe for Millie who has two jobs and five children to care for on her own.

A combination of all the above controls on the lives and health of the informants contributes to the degree of depression that they feel. For some, depression and worries are a major cause of ill-health. They can also act as a control on health because they form part of cycle that the informants find difficult to break. They suffer from depression which leads to more depression, and this adds to the worries that they also have. For some of the Asian informants this is particularly caused and exacerbated by their lack of English and, therefore, their isolation in Britain.

Another major influence on the health of the informants is fate or chance, or for the religious informants, God's will. Ill-health is accepted as just part of life, against which individuals are largely, with a few exceptions, powerless, and fate, chance or God's will are the controllers of who gets what illnesses, when. Another force the informants have to face is heredity. Although most agree that heredity exists, most would deny that it has any effects within their own families. There is a strong sense of fear amongst most of the informants that serious conditions could be passed on to them or their children from previous generations, and so it is considered best not to think too deeply about the chances of heredity in one's own family. They particularly fear life-threatening conditions such as cancer, stroke and the loss of function of any of the limbs or senses. A condition perceived to be less life-threatening and noticeable to others, however, such as sugar diabetes, is accepted by several to be hereditary within their own families. The type of condition, its effects and visibility to others may thus be an important factor in their beliefs about heredity.

The health-care services act as a control over the amount and quality of the treatment the informants receive when they are unwell. As shown in chapter three, the medical profession has some specific ideas about conditions it expects to find among black people, and it seems likely that doctors are also influenced by some of the material concerning racism and culture covered by chapters one and two. Among those interviewed, there was only one case of sickle-cell anaemia (Millie's son); one of thalassaemia-major (Sufiya's son); and one of tuberculosis (Tasneem). As mentioned in chapter three, these conditions are important and deserve attention from medical professionals, but they should not be the only focus of interest.

The action of specific doctors in determining who is entitled to treatment is also evident among the informants. Several of the Asians speak of occasions when they have been turned away by doctors who have claimed that they are exaggerating their complaints, or even that they have imagined them. This was so in respect of Tasneem's tuberculosis and in the others' experience of insensitive and unpleasant treatment where hospital personnel were rude or seemed to ignore them deliberately (such as Naseem's and Taresh's experiences in "E" hospital).

The informants of Afro-Caribbean descent also speak of occasions of doctors using their power to turn them away or to ignore their pains or discomfort. An obvious case is that of Millie and the contraceptive coil repeatedly fitted without her permission or knowledge, and without regard to her cultural practices. Millie also had experience of doctors refusing to treat her period pain because, she claimed, they had racist or sexist views. Judy was also refused treatment, and Carlton complained about insensitive treatment. The failure of Delores's doctor to diagnose her fibroids is another example, and one that could have resulted in serious problems if Delores had not been able to consult another doctor to arrange an emergency hysterectomy.

The control of doctors is also exhibited in the consulting room of the surgery. Many of the informants from both groups complain about their feelings of powerlessness in the face of doctors' knowledge and attitudes. These feelings are expressed particularly lucidly by Earl, Delores, Leroy and Taresh (chapters five and six). These opinions about professional power link clearly with the theories of professional dominance and assymetric power between patients and doctors examined in chapter two.

These, then, are powerful controls operating on the health of the informants. Some of these controls are clearly perceived by the informants to have important effects on their health; other controls are not so perceived. Despite their power, these controls do not entirely determine the levels of ill-health that are perceived or experienced by the informants. There are also the elements of context and choice which help, in some cases, to ameliorate the effects of some of the above controls.

Context

The events that surround the informants' lives can have important effects on their health and the ways in which they choose to react. On a large scale, their lives and health are clearly affected by the controls mentioned above, particularly the effects of the history of immigration and race relations in Britain. It is within the context of the history of immigration and race relations in Britain that this study is set. On a smaller scale, the specific context of particular episodes of ill-health will determine whether or not these episodes are ignored or perceived as illness or disease. Hence the informants may appear to hold contradictory beliefs or perceptions, but when the context is examined, reasons for the contradictions may be discovered. At one point in the interview, for example, the informant may say that she/he has never been ill, but then go on later to tell a story which describes one or more bouts of sometimes serious ill-health.

The effects of context on the larger scale has already been considered in the section on control, above, so this section will concentrate more on the importance and effects of context as it appears on the smaller scale. Here, the context becomes of crucial importance in determining whether a condition will be perceived as an illness in need of attention, an illness to be ignored, or not an illness at all. In some cases, the same condition with the same symptoms will be differentially perceived at different times, depending upon the context. Carlton, for example, recognised a cold as an illness when he was unemployed, but when he was working, colds were ignored and coped with as part of everyday life. Work has already been mentioned as a factor of great importance in the lives of the Afro-Caribbean informants who work, and work is often linked to a person's perceived state of health. The women of Asian descent who do not work feel that their lives are always affected by the context of their loss of friends and relatives when they migrated to Britain. Naseem, for example, makes it clear that this loss fills her with loneliness and depression that in turn make ill-health more likely. She thinks that if she were not lonely or depressed, she would be largely healthy.

The definition of a condition as an illness or a disease depends on the context within which the informant is thinking and acting. Martha, for example, when considering her experience of ill-health in her family, declares that she has never been ill, but when she compares herself with her workmates, she can see that her thyroid condition was a serious complaint. Some of the Asian informants, for example, when speaking of their ill-health as children, mention serious conditions such as smallpox and typhoid casually, because they were common, and yet they emphasise the importance of minor conditions such as headaches and 'flu that they experience now in Britain.

Episodes of ill-health must also be considered within the context in which they occur. A condition may be defined as an illness, but sympathy may be denied to the sufferer if she/he failed to take adequate precautions. Carlton, for example, blames his cold on playing football in the rain, and he does not really expect sympathy. Similarly, Naseem and Rani believe that if a person eats something which they know they are allergic to, they can only expect to become ill, and they will not, therefore, receive the same sort of sympathy as for a condition that "just happened".

Perceptions of ill-health may be influenced by recent occurrences. It is clear, for example, in the second interviews with Rani and Naseem that they have been affected by the shock of the stroke to their friend, Dalee. This is exhibited in their discussion of strokes as being illnesses they fear getting, and in their expression of shock as a cause of ill-health. Shobha reacts in a similar way to the deaths of her parents also by strokes. Some of the younger men of Afro-Caribbean descent have been similarly affected by media reports about sexually transmitted diseases. These effects emerge in their expression of their fears about getting herpes, VD or AIDS.

The informants' attitudes towards issues such as weight and smoking depend upon the context of their own experience. Most of the informants have read reports about the harmfulness to health of being overweight, for example, but not all of them believe the reports because they consider that they have been healthy while at the same time being, in medical terms, overweight. Some of the Afro-Caribbean informants feel that they are their "natural" weight, and they reject their GP's advice to diet. The attitude towards smoking is similar. Most of the Asian informants agree with reports that say that smoking is harmful to health because this fits in with their cultural and religious prohibitions on smoking. For some of the Afro-Caribbean informants, however, smoking marijuana is an important part of their culture, and so they cannot accept that smoking can be harmful to health.

The use of semi-structured, in-depth interviewing techniques allows an examination of the context of statements given by informants. The context is, in many cases, crucial to the interpretation of stories and statements about specific episodes of ill-health. On a larger scale, it is impossible to understand the state of health of black people without relating it to the wider context of the social, economic and political controls within which they live because these have a massive impact upon their lives, and ultimately, their health.

Choice

The health of the informants is not controlled entirely by the forces reported above. The personal and cultural heritages of the informants mean that they are able to make some choices as to what action to take. There is a link here between the patterns for behaviour outlined by cultural inheritance and the "recipes" for action postulated by Schutz (1972). The cultural heritage of the informants provide some recipes for action which are quite different from the western or professional medical options, and they also contain some traditional theories about how the body works. The amount of use made of these traditional cultural and family theories will depend on the context of the episode of ill-health and upon the degree of westernisation and the penetration of the professional medical ideology. The informants' backgrounds do allow them, however, a large range of choices.

"Culture", as described in chapter two, is the historical development of a group of people and contains their "recipes" for living in the world and coping with events such as ill-health (Saunders, 1954; Kroeber an Kluckholm, 1968). It has also been shown in chapter two that a person's cultural inheritance can affect her/his perceptions of health, expression and experience of symptoms, definitions of and responses to ill-health (Mechanic, 1978; Helman, 1978; Pfifferling, 1981). Cultural inheritance and family composition may determine the use of lay networks or non-professional healers as opposed to professional medical doctors (Dingwall, 1976; Mechanic, 1978; Pilisuk and Froland, 1978).

Typically, as shown in chapters one, two and three, "culture" has been seen by western observers to be a negative factor in black people's lives, and something which acts against their health. Cultural practices have, for example, been blamed for causing rickets and tuberculosis among Asians (BMJ, 1978; Galloway, 1965), and schizophrenia and child accidents among Afro-Caribbeans (Patterson, 1966; Littlewood and Lipsedge, 1982). Rarely, if ever, have beliefs and practices rooted in non-European cultures been examined positively. Yet it is clear from this research that the informants' cultural beliefs and practices may have beneficial effects on their health, and can be utilised in place of or alongside western medicine.

Several of the informants show, for example, that they do not share the western scientific view of how the body works. Using their own experiences and the ideas and theories handed down to them, they have worked out internally consistent theories which may not be "correct", but may beneficially affect their health. Joe and Delores are the principal West Indian theorists. Joe proffers an explanation for high rates of heart disease in Britain through his impression that the blood runs thicker in Britain. At another stage, Joe speaks of washing out the lungs with milk to prevent breathing in the dust at work. This is important, since he says that only recently have the bosses at work informed them that this dust is, in fact, asbestos, and he adds that unlike his other workmates, he has always taken care when handling dust.

Delores shares with several of the other Afro-Caribbean informants, theories about the flow of liquids in the body. The proper functioning of the blood circulation, menstrual cycle, digestive system and perspiration are all thought to be critical in the maintenance of good health. This has also been found by Kitzinger (1972; 1980). All of these things can be easily measured, and can be treated by home remedies, usually in the form of liquids. The use of remedies is one of the most important choices the Afro-Caribbean informants' culture affords. Most of them use at least herbal teas, and some use quite complicated compounds which are not always easy to obtain in Britain. The use of remedies and the reliance on the proper functioning of the liquids in the body means that the informants of Afro-Caribbean descent do not rely entirely on the NHS or private medical systems. They choose when to use either. Typically, home remedies will be tried first, and then if the condition remains or worsens after three days or so, GPs may be consulted, depending upon the severity and context of the episode.

The informants of Asian descent do not have the same sort of range of home remedies or theories about the workings of the body as those of Afro-Caribbean descent, but some cultural ideas remain. They speak, for example, about the importance of temperature, particularly the balancing of hot and cold forces in the body. The perception of some episodes of ill-health as hot or cold allows them to select the sort of food which should restore balance. The traditional theories are not always referred to, however, because they are quite different to the theories operated by the informants' GPs, and usually the context of the episode will prove to be crucial here.

The informants of Asian descent have similar attitudes towards the old theories about weight. Some still believe that to be fat is healthy, and these are, typically, the ones who are overweight, such as Dalee. Others hold to the modern ideas and want to be slim; and still others use both theories, depending on the context. Tasneem, for example, wants to be slim herself, but she also wants her children to be quite fat so that they look healthy to her friends, and because, deep down, she still believes in the traditional theories.

A choice that many of the informants make is to be religious. For the informants of Asian descent, this means that their lives are structured for them around the times of prayer, particular practices and in the advocacy of things such as cleanliness and purity. Their religions also help to give them a sense of purpose in their lives, and give a great sense of contentment and strength to cope with the loneliness they feel and the ill-health they suffer. Their religions, therefore, affect their mental health positively, and can also have effects on their physical health by preventing the eating of foods which are thought to cause certain illnesses or diseases, or habits known to be harmful to health such as smoking. There are, inevitably, some harmful effects, such as the much vaunted lack of vitamin D in the traditional diet, but on the whole, the average Asian diet is thought by nutritionists to be much healthier than the average British diet (see chapter three).

Many of the informants of Afro-Caribbean descent also choose to follow religions, and they also gain great strength to cope with the unpleasantnesses of everyday life. Many times they speak of reading the bible or praying which, they say, alleviate the burden of worries and depression they carry and ease them through the tasks they have to perform. Some of the women attend healing churches, where specific episodes of ill-health are seen to be cured through faith and the laying on of hands. Religion can be seen to be both a control and a choice: a control because it is an integral part of culture and limits activities; and a choice because individuals can decide to select only certain parts of it for their own convenience, or to discard it altogether.

The Afro-Caribbean informants who do not rely on religion take instead to sport. Exercise and sport, the young men believe, may help to increase their lifespan and help to keep their bodies in good physical shape. Sport can help, they think, in toughening up the body's natural defences, but it can also lead to some weaknesses. Paul says, for example, that there is always a period of vulnerability to germs just after a hard game of football. Most of the other informants agree with the young men about the value to health of exercise, but few have the time or inclination to practise what they believe.

In chapters five and six, the informants made it clear that they thought food was an important determinant of good health. The choice of food can, therefore, affect a person's health. Several of the informants of both groups still eat their traditional diets, but sometimes this becomes difficult owing to the limited availability of tropical produce, or the expense of it, and so some substitution does occur. Many of the informants now eat, or at least prepare for their children, western-style dishes, and many have absorbed "junk" food into their diets. The nutritional effects of this seem, as yet, uninvestigated, although it is probable that rates of heart disease are rising to typical western levels amongst people of Asian or Afro-Caribbean descent.

Health education has attacked the traditional diets of people of Asian descent as part of its policy, and some of this criticism has reached and affects the informants. Several of the Asians spoke about not knowing any more what they should eat and how it should be prepared. Some find it difficult to cope with husbands who demand traditional foods and children who demand western dishes such as beef burgers. Tasneem says she has adopted an almost totally western diet, mainly because her doctors told her that Asian diets are bad for health. Despite the intense propaganda to try to convince Asians that they should use margarine rather than butter in order to raise their levels of vitamin D, many of the informants still use butter and other dairy products because these are central to their theories of the value of food. There are some, however, who now use margarine, and some who have used it for some time out of preference.

The informants of Afro-Caribbean descent have not been the specific target for any health education about diet. Most of the older informants still prefer their traditional dishes, although some, like Martha, make them very rarely now. Most of the younger informants have taken to eating what they call "conventional" food - a totally western diet, although they have fond memories of the food their mothers cooked. Carlton, who lives at home, considers traditional food to be the major source of his strength and the reason he can outrun all his white friends. Leroy and Earl have moved over to western diet because their girlfriends are white and they seem quite happy to do so.

As far as the health services are concerned, the informants can choose which practitioners they use and when. The informants of Asian descent, for example, can choose between a male or female, white or Asian GP depending on the advice of others and on their perceived needs. Some of those who speak little English derive much comfort from being able to express their worries in their chosen language. The informants of Afro-Caribbean descent are willing to consult private doctors if they are not satisfied with their NHS GPs, and those who do add that they are used to paying for health care in the Caribbean. The stories told, for example by Delores, seem to support their feeling of a need for a second opinion. The Afro-Caribbeans also express their skepticism of GPs by not consulting them unless they have to.

There are several instances in the interviews where doctors would have been much more useful to the informants if they had been aware of the informants' cultural practices or principles. Their prescription of drugs, for example, would be much more effective and accurate if they were aware that some of their patients preferred liquid preparations or felt that too many western drugs were bad for their health. Similarly, Millie could have been spared much anguish and ill-health if doctors had been sensitive to her cultural practice of not having intercourse for up to six months after the birth of her baby, and had later explained about the contraceptive coil that they forced her to accept.

The use of in-depth interviews, the ability to probe answers and to cross-check information has allowed the emergence of parts of the informants' cultural heritage. Cultural practices and beliefs may be different from scientific practices and theories, but that does not automatically mean that they are injurious to health or that they are so unimportant that they can be ignored. What is important is that the people who hold theories and ideas are likely to use them, and so ignorance of, and insensitivity to them is often the cause of anguish and unnecessary pain. In some cases, cultural practices may cause actual harm, but in others they provide a range of choices for the informants which can have beneficial effects on their health. The insidious invasion of western ideology is evident in some of the responses of the informants, but it is also true that despite this, some aspects of culture remain intact and are utilised.

Conclusion

The lives of the informants are largely controlled by factors outside their own influence. These include the workings of the labour and property markets which tend to concentrate black people into certain sectors and areas. Racism is an expression of these controls and has helped to maintain the low political, social and economic position of black people - workers and non-workers. Inside these overarching constraints, it has been shown that the informants are able and willing to make some choices which can affect their everyday lives. These choices, such as the practising of remedies and the following of religious beliefs and practice, do not alter the structure of their lives, but they are perceived to make their lives seem more bearable.

The methodology of the project has helped to illuminate these factors, and stress the importance of context. In any study of black people, the larger context of immigration and race relations in Britain must be taken into account if individual lives are to be understood. At a smaller scale, it has been shown that the context of people's perceptions and statements about their health and lives can be crucial to an adequate and accurate understanding of their lives. Opinions taken out of context may, for example, lead to distorted views of what individuals meant at particular times and places.

This chapter began with an account of the similarities and differences between the two groups of informants in their attitudes towards health, ill-health and the health services. It went on to link these attitudes to the introductory chapters on race relations, culture, health research and the methodology of the study. It has concluded with the observations that the lives and health of the informants depend largely on societal constraints over which they have little, if any, control, but within which they are able to exercise a few, albeit minor, choices of action; and that any attempts to understand their perceptions and attitudes towards health matters must take into account they contexts (on large and small scales) within which their everyday lives are played out.

BLACK PEOPLE'S HEALTH : A CONCLUSION

The aim of this project has been to examine and understand the perceptions and experiences of health, ill-health and the health services of two groups of people of Asian and Afro-Caribbean descent. In attempting to fulfil this aim, the study has been set within the context of the history of immigration and race-relations in Britain since the second world war. Within this large scale context, a definition of "culture" has been sought, and its effects on perceptions of health considered. The debate on the primacy of culture or race as the explanatory variable in black people's health has also been investigated, as has the body of literature associated with ethnicity and health. In an attempt to take a different approach from the bulk of this literature, the methodology of the study was developed out of the ethnographic and interpretative sociological traditions. In this way, the emphasis in the empirical work has been on the wholeness and uniqueness of thirty individual case-studies, and the interpretations and views of the world of the informants have been taken to be paramount.

Some of the findings of the empirical work replicate those of Cornwell (1984). There is some evidence of, for example, the existence of private and public accounts of life events. Public accounts are views of illnesses, family relationships and so on that are acceptable to outsiders, that may not be the "truth", but are representations of an image that people wish to project about themselves. Private accounts, however, are closer to the "truth", and are usually divulged during the telling of stories about particular events and episodes in their lives. Hence people generally say that they like and are satisfied with the treatment they receive from their GP (a public account), but may go on at a later stage to describe specific objections to and complaints about the same GP (a private account).

The distinction between private and public accounts is an attractive one, but it may not be the only explanation of people's contradictory attitudes. It can be seen, for example, that individuals may hold and express positive views of doctors in general, but complain about one GP in particular. Similarly, one unpleasant experience of treatment by a GP may not alter the individual's overall positive image of the doctor or doctors in general. People seem quite able to hold apparently contradictory views about the same thing. It may be that the most important factor is the context within which they are speaking. Persisting with the same example, talking in general about "doctors" will produce a positive statement, but when the discussion is shifted to the incident of unpleasant treatment, a negative view is likely to be expressed.

The importance of the context or public and private accounts of contradictory views emphasises the value of the chosen methodology. It is only when people are allowed and encouraged to tell stories about their experiences that they divulge the context within which they are speaking and/or their private accounts. Consequently, traditional social surveys, with their emphasis on fitting people's opinions into a few categories, miss the wealth of detail which helps to explain why people hold particular views at particular times.

The analysis of the wealth of material produced by the semi-structured interviews has also provided important evidence for the refutation of many stereotypes currently held about black people and which have been shown to be operating against some of the informants. The conceptions, for example, that Asian family life is dominated by an autocratic male, that arranged marriages must be unhappy and that Asian women cannot stand pain and only want to see female doctors, do not hold as far as these informants are concerned. Similarly, theories about "uncaring" Afro-Caribbean one-parent families and the "criminality" of black youth can also be rejected. Such stereotypes are not only incorrect, but they affect how black people are treated by professionals and in general. Stereotyping is an insidious form of racism.

This thesis has, then, attempted to examine and understand the perceptions and experiences of health, ill-health and the health care services of thirty informants of Afro-Caribbean and Asian descent. The ethnographical approach has emphasised the importance of the informants' points of view and the meanings that they attach to things in their everyday lives. The context has been shown to be important, both in the wider sense of the history of immigration and race relations, and in the narrower sense of the events surrounding individual perceptions of episodes of ill-health or other life events. The study has shown the inappropriateness and biased nature of much of the previous research in ethnicity and health, particularly that which concentrates on unusual conditions or on cultural/ethnic "explanations" for disease occurrences. The project has also exposed the unreliability and often racist nature of stereotypes held about black people or their families. Most critically, perhaps, the study has contributed to the debate on the primacy of racism or culture, finding that the informants' lives are largely controlled by social, economic and political systems which act against them owing to the structural position imposed on them because of the colour of their skin.

APPENDICES

APPENDIX I

Points For The Lifestory Interviews

This appendix contains the questions which were generally, but not always, put to the informants during the first interview which was concerned with eliciting details of their life- and health-histories. The order of the questions was largely determined by the responses of individual informants; the listing below is merely an indication of the sorts of questions used. Points marked with an asterisk were asked only of women - they concern issues of pregnancy and menstruation - and bracketed questions were asked of the Asian women - they concern issues of language.

Childhood

Where were you brought up?
Were you a healthy child?
What illnesses/diseases do you remember having?
Who looked after you when you were ill?
Did you ever see a doctor or some other healer?
Did you ever go to hospital?
Did your family have any particular ways to stay in good health?
or any home remedies for certain illnesses?

Adolescence

Where did you live during your teenage years?
Were you healthy then?
When did you leave .... ?
What was that experience like?
*Can you remember when your periods started?
*Any trouble since?
*How many pregnancies have you had?
*Were you healthy during them?
*What was the first pregnancy like?
*Did you go to ante-natal classes?
*Who delivered your babies? And where?

Present health

How would you describe your health at the moment?

Can you remember the last time you felt unwell? What was wrong? What were its symptoms? What did you do? What caused it? Did it worry you?

Is your health important to you?

Have you ever been seriously ill?

Do you have any illnesses that keep coming back?

Do you smoke cigarettes? Some people say that smoking is bad for health - do you agree or disagree?

Is exercise important for good health?

Have you taken any medicine, tablets or ointments recently? What are they? Do they work?

Do you prefer to take tablets or medicines, or do you not mind either?

Do you take vitamin tablets or tonics?

Do you ever get depressed?

Family

- Ask about the health of husband/wife/partner and any children

Is there anything about the health of anyone in your family that worries you?

Health services

- Ask about NHS GP - registered? how did you choose the doctor? how long have you had this doctor?

- And the surgery - happy with it? appointments?

Are you satisfied with this/these doctor/s?

What do you like about her/him/them?

[Do you need to take a friend or relative as an interpreter? Is this OK?]

Have you ever been asked to pay for anything at the doctor's?

Tell me about the last time you saw the doctor - what was it for? etc.

Do doctors treat everybody the same?

Are the drugs doctors prescribe better than home remedies?

Have you ever been to hospital? When was the last time? What for? etc.

Have you been to A&E? What for? etc.

Where is the nearest hospital doing A&E? Have you been there?

Are there any other hospitals around here? Have you ever been to them?

What do you think of the NHS?

Have you ever been to a private doctor [or hakim]? What for? etc. How did you choose her/him? Value for money?

Is there anyone who is not a doctor who you would talk to about illness?

Have there been any times recently when you've felt like going to see a doctor, but in the end you didn't bother? What was wrong? etc.

<u>Race, sex and class</u>

Are you working at the moment? What do you do?

Do you like working, or would you prefer to be at home? Or vice-versa, if applicable.

Do you think your work/being at home could have any effects on your health?

Is your partner/wife/husband working, or your children?

Do you think his/their work could have any effects on their health?

Do you think you've ever been treated differently because you're black?

*Or because you're a woman?

Are you a religious person?

Can religion help people at all?

Are you happy living here?

Has living in Britain/London affected your health?

What do you think about the government? The police? Your/your children's education?

What do you think your health will be like in the future?

And your/your children's life/lives?

APPENDIX II

Issues for the Second Round

Is there any such thing as perfect health? Have you got it?

Should everyone expect to be ill, sometime?

Can you do anything to stop yourself getting ill?

What, for you, is an illness?

Is there any difference between an illness and a disease?

Do germs exist/cause illnesses?

Have you heard of viruses?

Is your body naturally resistant to germs/viruses?

Do some illnesses/diseases run in the family?

Can loneliness cause illnesses?

Can tiredness cause illnesses?

Can where you work affect your health?

Can where you live affect your health?

Can unemployment affect your health?

Is it ever anybody's fault when they get ill? Has it ever been your fault?

Can a shock cause ill-health/make it worse?

Can racial discrimination cause ill-health? How does it affect you?

Is it inevitable that children will get measles etc?

Are there any illnesses/diseases that it is inevitable adults will get?

Are there any illnesses/diseases you are afraid of getting?

Are there any incurable conditions? Why do some people get them?

Are there any illnesses/diseases that you remember people used to get that they don't seem to get these days?

What are the first signs that you are ill?

How important is temperature?

Are there hot and cold illnesses/diseases?

How important are the concepts hot and cold to you?

If you are ill, should you avoid certain foods or drinks?

Who is healthier, a fat person or a slim one?

Are religious people more likely to be healthy than non-believers?

Do you use home remedies at all?

Bibliography

Abbreviations

Am = American	Hum = Human
Behav = Behaviour	J = Journal
B/Br = British	M = Medical
CHGEM = Community Health Group for Ethnic Minorities	Med = Medicine
Contemp = Contemporary	Prev = Preventative
Educ = Education	Proc = Proceedings
Epid = Epidemiology	Prog = Progress
Gen = General	Sci = Science
Geog = Geography	Serv = Services
Hlth = Health	Soc = Social/Society
Hosp = Hospital	Trans = Transactions
	Uni = University

Agar, M. H. 1980 The Professional Stranger, Academic Press, London.

Aho, W.R. & Minott, K. 1977 Creole and doctor medicine, Social Science and Medicine, 11, 349-355.

Alexander, B 1974 Help for immigrant families, Nursing Times, 70, 17.

Ali, A.R. et al 1978 Surma and lead poisoning, BMJ, 2, 915-6.

Allen, S. 1982 in Husband, op.cit, 128-144.

Allen, S. & Smith, C. 1974 in Parkin, F. (ed) The Social Analysis of Class Structure, Tavistock, London.

Anionwu, E. & Beattie, A. 1981 Learning to cope, Nursing Times, July 8th, 1214-1219.

Anwar, M. 1979 The Myth of Return, Heineman, London.

Apple, D. 1960 How laymen define illness, J. Health and Human Behaviour, 1, 219-25.

Arneil, G.C. & Crosbie, J.C. 1963 Infantile rickets in Glasgow, The Lancet, 2, ii, 423-5.

Aslam, M. et al 1979 Compliance in medication, Nursing Times, 75, 22, 931-2.

Aslam, M. et al 1981 In the best of traditions? Nursing Mirror, 153, 4, 134-6

Aslam, M. & Davis, S.S. 1980 The hakim and his role, Report to the DHSS, OHMS.

Aslam, M. & Stockley, I.H. 1979 Karela and drug interactions, The Lancet, 1, 607.

Atkinson, P. 1981 The Clinical Experience, Gower, London.

Bagley, C. 1968 Migration, race and mental health, Race, IX, 3, 343-56.

Ballard, R. 1982 in Rapoport and Rapoport (eds), Families in Britain, Routledge and Kegan Paul, London, 179-204.

Banton, M. 1967 Race Relations, Tavistock, London.

Banton, M. 1977 The Idea of Race, Tavistock, London.

Baran, P.A. & Sweezy, P.M. 1966 Monopoly Capital, Penguin, Harmondsworth.

Barker, M. 1981 The New Racism, Junction Books, London.

Barron, S.L. & Vessey, M 1966 Birthweight of infants, B.J. Prev. & Soc. Med., 20, 127-134

Bebbington, P.E. 1978 Epidemiology of depressive disorder, Culture, Medicine and Psychiatry, 2, 297-341.

Becker, H.S. et al 1961 Boys in White, Uni. Chicago Press, Chicago.

Bell, C. & Newby, H. (eds) 1977 Doing Sociological Research, George Allen & Unwin, London.

Ben-Tovim, G. et al 1982 in Husband, op.cit., 301-324.

Berger, P. & Kellner, H. 1970 Marriage and the construction of reality, in Dreitzel, op.cit., 50-72.

Berger, P. & Luckman, T. 1966 The Social Construction of Reality, Allen Lane, London.

Bernstein, R.J. 1976 The Restructuring of Social and Political Theory, Blackwell, Oxford.

Black Health Workers & Patients Group 1983 Psychiatry and the corporate state, Race and Class, XXV, 2, 49-63.

Blaxter, M. 1983 Causes of disease, Social Science and Medicine, 17, 2, 59-69.

Blumer, H. 1962 Society as symbolic interaction, in Rose, op.cit., 179-92.

Bourne, J. & Sivanandan, A. 1980 Cheerleaders and Ombudsmen, Race and Class, 21, 4, 331-351.

Bowden, C.L. & Burnstein, A.G. 1979 Psychological basis of medical practice, Williams and Williams, Baltimore.

Brass, T 1983 in the Sunday Times, 6th January.

Brearley, P. et al 1978 The Social Context of Health-Care, Martin Robertson, London.

Brent Community Health Council	1981	Black People and the Health Service, Brent Community Health Council, London.
Br.J.Prev. & Soc. Med.	1977	Editorial, Br.J. Prev. & Soc. Med., 27.
BMJ	1975	Editorial: Sickle Cell disease, BMJ, 2
BMJ	1978	Editorial: Rickets, BMJ, 1, B
BMJ	1979	Editorial: Rickets, BMJ, 6180, 1744.
BMJ	1980	Editorial: Paranoia, BMJ, 281
BMJ	1981	Editorial: Ethnic factors in disease, BMJ, 282, 1496-7.
Brody, H. (ed)	1981	Ethical Decisions in Medicine, Little, Brown & Co, Boston.
Brooks, O.G. et al	1981	Intra-uterine Vitamin D, BMJ, 283.
Brown, C.	1984	Black and White Britain: The Third PSI Survey, Heinemann, London.
Burgess, E.W.	1927	Case studies as methods, Sociology and Social Research, XII, 2 103-20.
Burgess, R. (ed)	1982	Field Research: A Sourcebook and Field Manual, George Allen & Unwin, London.
Burghe, P.L. van den	1978	Race and Racism, John Wiley, London.
Burke, A.W.	1976	Attempted suicide, Br. J. Psychiatry, 128, 528-33.
Bynner, J. & Stribley, K. (eds)	1978	Social Research, Longman, London.
Carby, H.V.	1982a	in CCCS, op.cit., 183-211.
Carby, H.V.	1982b	in CCCS, op.cit., 212-235.
Carne, S.	1970	Immigrant patient, Proc. Royal Soc. Med., 63.
Carter, C.O. & Peel, J.	1976	Equalities and Inequalities in Health, Academic Press, London.
Cartwright, A.	1967	Patients and Their Doctors, Routledge and Kegan Paul, London.
Castles, S. & Kosack, G.	1973	Immigrant Workers and Class Structure in Western Europe, OUP, London.
Centre for Contemporary Cultural Studies (CCCS)	1982	The Empire Strikes Back, Hutchinson, London.
Cicourel, A.V.	1964	Method and Measurement in Sociology, Collier-Macmillan, London.

Clarke, C., Ley, D. & Peach, C. (eds)	1984	Geography and Ethnic Pluralism, George Allen and Unwin, London.
Clarke, M et al	1979	Tuberculosis mortality, Community Medicine, 1, 23-8.
Clyne, M.B.	1976	Racial and cultural factors of relevance for the GP, Proc. Royal Soc. Med., 69, 635-7.
Coard, B.	1971	How the West Indian Child is Made Educationally Sub-Normal, New Beacon Books, London.
Cochrane, R. et al	1977	Measuring psychological disturbance in Asian immigrants, Soc. Sci. & Med., 11, 157-64.
Cochrane, R.	1979a	Psychological and behavioural disturbance, Medical News, 11, 6, 2.
Cochrane, R.	1979b	Psychological disturbance, Br. J. Psychiatry, 134, 201-10.
Cochrane, R. & Stopes-Roe, M.	1980	The mental health of immigrants, New Community, 8, 123-8.
Coe, R.M.	1978	Sociology of Medicine, McGraw-Hill, New York.
Cohen, A.	1974	Urban Ethnicity, Tavistock, London.
Colfax, J.D.	1971	Varieties and prospects of "radical scholarship" in Colfax & Roach, op.cit., 81-92.
Colfax, J.D. & and Roach, J.L. (eds)	1971	Radical Sociology, Basic Books, New York.
Commission for Racial Equality (CRE)	1984	Race and Council Housing in Hackney, CRE, London.
Community Relations Commission	1976	Mental Health among Minority Groups, CRC, London.
Contemporary Issues in Geog. and Educ.	1984	Geography and Education for a Multicultural Society, Contemp. Issues in Geog and Educ. 1, 2, 1-2.
Cooke, W.T. et al	1974	Rickets and growth, BMJ, 2, 293-7.
Cooper, R. et al	1981	Racism, society and disease, Internat. J. of Health Services, II, 3, 389-414.

Cooper, R. 1983 Race and the social origins of disease, Radical Community Medicine, 16, Winter, 5-19.

Cornwell, J. 1984 Hard-Earned Lives, Tavistock, London.

Cottle, T.J. 1978 Black Testimony, Wildwood House, London.

Cox, C. & Mead, A. (eds) 1975 A Sociology of Medical Practice, Collier Macmillan, London.

Cox, J. 1980 Deprivation in minority ethnic groups, MIMS magazine, 1st May, 35-41.

Cox, O.C. 1948 Caste, Class and Race, Monthly Review Press, New York.

Croog, S.H. 1961 Ethnic origins and responses to health questionnaire, Human Organisation, 20, 2, 65-9.

Cruikshank, J.K. et al 1980 Heart attack, stroke, diabetes, and hypertension in West Indians, Asians and whites in Birmingham, BMJ, 281, 1108.

Culyer, A.J. 1976 Need and the NHS, Martin Robertson, London.

Dahya, B. 1974 in Cohen, A. (ed), Urban Ethnicity, Tavistock, London, 77-118.

Daily Mail 1978 Report of speech of M. Thatcher, 31st January.

Danna, J.J. 1980 Migration and mental health, Culture, Medicine and Psychiatry, 4, 25-42.

Davie, E. 1979 The cultural dimension, Community Care, 264, 36-9.

Davis, L.R. et al 1981 Survey of sickle-cell disease in England and Wales, BMJ, 283, 1519-21.

Davis, S.S. & Aslam, M. 1979 Eastern treatment for Eastern health? J. Community Nursing, 2, 11, 16-20.

Davis, S.S. & Aslam, M. 1980 The Hakim and his role, Rept to DHSS, London

Deakin, N. 1970 in Zubaida, op.cit., 17-34.

Denzin, N.K. 1978 The Research Act, McGraw-Hill, New York.

DHSS 1980a The Black Report: Inequalities in Health, HMSO, London.

DHSS 1980b Rickets and Osteomalacia, HMSO, London.

Dingwall, R. 1976 Aspects of Illness, Martin Robertson, London.

Dodge, J 1971 Impact of immigration on medicine, Br.J. Hosp. Med., 5, 1, 47-50.

Donovan, J.L. 1982 Ethnicity and Health, Dept. of Geography Working Paper No. 3, QMC.

Donovan, J.L. 1983 Black people's health: a different way forward, Radical Community Medicine, Winter, 20-29.

Donovan. J.L. 1984 Ethnicity and Health, Social Science & Medicine, 19, 7, 663-70.

Donovan, J.L. 1985 Black Women's Health, Middlesex Poly Occasional Paper, forthcoming.

Douglas, J. (ed) 1971 Understanding Everyday Life, Routledge and Kegan Paul, London.

Doyal, L. 1979 Political Economy of Health, Pluto, London.

Doyal, L. 1983 Cancer in Britain, Pluto, London.

Doyal, L. et al 1980 Migrant Workers in the NHS, Dept. Sociology, Poly of N. London, SSRC.

Dreitzel, H.P. 1970 Recent Sociology, Macmillan, New York.

Driver, G. 1982 in Rapoport and Rapoport (eds) op.cit., 205-219.

Dunnell, K. & Cartwright, A. 1972 Medicine Takers, Prescribers and Hoarders, Routledge and Kegan Paul, London.

Durkeim, E. 1938 The Rules of Sociological Method, Free Press, Illinois.

Durkeim, E. 1952 Suicide, Routledge & Kegan Paul, London.

Durkeim, E. et al 1960 Essays on Sociology and Philosophy, Harper & Row, New York.

Eagle, R. 1980 Your friendly neighbourhood hakim, World Medicine, 15, 21, 19-22.

Easterday, L. 1982 The making of a female researcher, in Burgess, op.cit., 62-7.

Eckstein, H. 1975 Case study theory, in Greenstein, F. & Polsby, N. (eds) Handbook of Political Science, vol 7, Addison-Wesley, Mass.

Ehrenreich, J. (ed) 1978 The Cultural Crisis of Modern Medicine, Monthly Review Press, New York.

Eisenberg, L. 1977 Disease and illness, Culture, Medicine and Psychiatry, 1, 9-23.

Eisenberg, L. 1980 What makes persons patients, Am. J. of Medicine, 69, 277-286.

Eisenberg, L. & Kleinman, A. (eds) 1981 The Relevance of Social Science for Medicine, D. Reidel, Dordrecht.

Emerson, P.A. & Beath, G. 1961 Tuberculosis in Soho, BMJ, 2, 148-52.

Enos, D.D. & Sultan, P. 1977 The Sociology of Health Care, Praeger, New York.

Epstein, A.L. (ed) 1967 The Craft of Social Anthropology, Tavistock, London.

Evans, P. 1971 Attitudes of Young Immigrants, Runnymede Trust, London.

Eyles, J.D. 1974 Social theory and social geography, Prog. in Geog., 6, 27-87.

Eyles, J.D. & Woods, K. 1983 A Social Geography of Health, Croom Helm, London.

Fabrega, H. 1977 The scope of ethnomedical science, Culture, Medicine and Psychiatry, 1, 201-228.

Fabrega, H. & Tyma, S. 1976 Culture, language and the shaping of illness, J. of Psychosomatic Research, 20, 232-237.

Fanon, F. 1963 The Wretched of the Earth, Penguin, Harmondsworth.

Fernyhough, D. 1979 Culture colours diagnosis, British Medicine, 21st June, 6-8.

Ferreyra, C. 1981 Politics and Ethnic Minority Health, CHGEM, London.

Feyerabend, P.K. 1970 Against Method, Uni. of Minnesota Press, Minnesota.

Filmer, P. et al 1972 New Directions in Sociological Theory, Collier-Macmillan, London.

Foner, N. 1979 Jamaica Farewell, Routledge and Kegan Paul, London.

	1977	Fontana Dictionary of Modern Thought, Collins, London.
Foot, P.	1965	Immigration and Race in British Politics, Penguin, Harmondsworth.
Ford, J.A. et al	1972a	Rickets and osteomalacia, BMJ, 2, 211-12.
Ford, J.A. et al	1972b	Biochemical response of late rickets, BMJ, 2, 677-80.
Ford, J.A. et al	1973	Neonatal rickets, BMJ, 3, A, 446-7.
Freidson, E.	1970a	Professional Dominance, Atherton Press, New York.
Freidson, E.	1970b	Profession of Medicine, Dodd Mead & Co, New York
Freidson, E.	1975	in Cox, C. and Mead, A. A Sociology of Medical Practice, Collier-Macmillan, London.
Fryer, P.	1984	Staying Power, Pluto Press, London.
Galloway, J	1965	Immigration in the Midlands, The Lancet, 2, 731-2.
Ganathe, N.S.	1981	Learn Urdu Through English, Balaji, Madras.
Gans, B	1966	in Wolstenholme, G & O'Connor, M, Immigration: Social and Medical Aspects, Churchill, London, 85-93.
Garfinkel, H.	1967	Studies in Ethnomethodology, Prentice Hall, New Jersey.
Garner, L.	1979	Your Money or Your Life, Penguin, Harmondsworth.
Giddens, A.	1976	New Rules of Sociological Method, Hutchinson, London.
Gill, D.	1983	Education for a multiracial society, Contemp. Issues in Geog. and Educ., 1, 1, 21-25.
Gilroy, P.	1980	Managing the underclass, Race and Class, XXII, 1, 47-62.
Gilroy, P.	1982	in CCCS, op.cit., 143-182.
Glaser, B.G. & Strauss, A.L.	1967	The Discovery of Grounded Theory, Aldine, Chicago.
Glendenning, F	1980	Another turn of the screw, New Age, Spring, 27-9.

Gluckman, M. 1961 Ethnographic data, Sociological Review, 9, 1, 5-26.

Goel, K.M. et al 1976 Florid and sub-clinical rickets, The Lancet, 1, ii, 1141-5.

Goel, K.M. et al 1981 Reduced prevalence of rickets, The Lancet, 2, 8243, 405-6.

Good, B.J. & Good, M.J. 1981 in Eisenberg & Kleinman, op.cit., 165-196.

Gordon, E.B. 1965 Mentally ill West Indians, Br.J. Psychiatry, 111, 877-87.

Gorman, R.A. 1975 Alfred Schutz, Br. J. Sociology, 26, 1, 1-19.

Gould, P. & White, R. 1974 Mental Maps, Penguin, Harmondsworth.

Graham, H. 1982 Building a Feminist Methodology, Brit. Sociological Assoc. Conf. Paper.

Greater London Council 1980 Social Review of Greater London, Social Policy Group, GLC.

Greater London Council 1982 The NHS and Ethnic Minorities, Ethnic Minorities Unit, London

Greenstein, F. & Polsby, N. (eds) 1975 Handbook of Political Science, Vol 8, Addison-Wesley, Mass.

Guardian 1984 Housing Allocation Review, The Guardian, 13th January, p4.

Guardian 1984 Sherman, A., 15th February.

Habermas, J. 1971 Toward a Rational Society, Heinemann, London.

Hackney CHC 1981 Advising Asian mothers, Hlth. & Soc. Ser. J., Oct 9th, 1244-5.

Hall, S. 1978 in Lane, D. et al (eds), Five Views of Multi-Racial Britain, CRE and BBC, London, 23-35.

Hall, S. et al 1978 Policing the Crisis, Macmillan, London.

Hammersley, M. & Atkinson, P. 1983 Ethnography, Tavistock, London.

Hannay, D.R. 1979 The Symptom Iceberg, Routledge and Kegan Paul, London.

Hashmi, F. 1966 in Wolstenholme, G. op.cit.

Hashmi, F. 1970 Immigrants and emotional stress, Proc. Royal Soc. Med., 63, 629-36.

Hlth & Soc. Ser. J. 1978 Editorial, Hlth. & Soc. Ser. J., 88.

Health Research Group 1982 Contemporary Perspectives on Health and Health Care, Occ. Paper 20, Dept. Geog. QMC.

Helman, C,G, 1978 Feed a cold, starve a fever, Culture, Medicine and Psychiatry, 2, 107-37.

Helman, C.G. 1984 Culture, Health and Illness, Wright, Bristol.

Herbert, D.T. & Smith, D.M. (eds) 1979 Social Problems and the City, OUP, Oxford.

Herzlich, C. 1973 Health and Illness, Academic Press, London.

Hicks, D. 1982 Review of bias in geography textbooks, Centre of Multicultural Education, London Institute of Education.

Hill, C. 1970 Immigration and Integration, Pergamon Press, Oxford.

Hindess, B. 1972 The "phenomenological" sociology of Schutz, Economy & Society, 1, 1, 1-27.

Hiro, D. 1973 Black British, White British, Monthly Review Press, London.

Hirst, P.Q. 1976 Social Evaluation & Sociological Categories, George Allen & Unwin, London.

Hitch, P. 1981 Immigrants and mental health, New Community, 9, 2.

Homans, H. & Satow, A. 1981 We too are strangers, J. Community Nursing, 5, 5, 10-13.

Hsu, F.L.K. 1955 in Paul, op.cit., 135-154.

Hunt, S.M. et al 1981 Nottingham health profile, Soc. Sci. & Med., 15A, 3, 221-9.

Husband, C. (ed) 1982 "Race" in Britain, Hutchinson, London.

Illich, I. 1976 Medical Nemesis, Penguin, Harmondsworth.

Ingham, M 1981 Impressions of mental and emotional health among Bengali women, Unpub. MSc dissert, Bedford Coll., London.

Inner London Educ Auth 1983 Race, Sex and Class, ILEA, London.

Jackson, P. & Smith, S.	1984	Exploring Social Geography, George Allen and Unwin, London.
Jt. TB Committee	1978	TB among immigrants, BMJ, 1, 6119, 1038-40.
Jones, C.	1977	Immigration and Social Policy in Britain, Tavistock, London.
Jordan, W.D.	1982	in Husband, op.cit., 42-58.
Kapo, R.	1981	A Savage Culture, Quartet, London.
Keil, J.E. et al	1980	Hypertension in Southall, J. Epid. & Community Hlth, 34, 45-7.
Keohane, N. et al (eds)	1979	Feminist Theory, Harvester, London.
Khan, V.S.	1977	in Watson, op.cit., 57-89.
Khan, V.S. (ed)	1979	Minority Families in Britain, Macmillan, London.
Khan, V.S.	1982	in Husband, op.cit., 197-215.
Khogali, M	1979	TB among immigrants, J.Epid. & Community Health, 33, 2, 134.
Kiev, A.	1963	Beliefs and delusions of West Indian immigrants, Br. J. Psychiatry, 109, 356-63.
Kiev, A	1964	Psychiatric illness among West Indians, Race, V, 3, 48-54.
King, J.	1982	How we see illness, New Society, 59, 1008, 388-9.
King, S.J.	1962	Perceptions of illness and Medical Practice, Russell Sage, New York.
Kitzinger, S.	1972	Body fantasies, New Society, 21, 510, 12-13.
Kitzinger, S.	1980	How the West Indies work, Gen. Practitioner, 15th Feb, 56-9.
Klein, R.	1979	Using the wrong label, Mind Out, 33, 16-18.
Kleinman, A.M.	1977	Depression, somatisation and new cross-cultural psychiatry, Soc. Sci. & Med., 11, 3-10.
Kleinman, A.	1980	Patients and Healers in the Context of Culture, Uni. California Press, London.
Kleinman, A., Good, B. & Eisenberg, M.D.	1978	Culture, illness and care, Annals of Internal Medicine, 88, 251-58.

Knight, L. 1979 Eastern promise in the East End, Nursing Mirror, 149, 17, 35-7.

Knight, L. 1981 Racism is a number one health problem, Mind Out, 41, 3-4.

Knox-Macaulay, H.et al 1973 Thalassaemia in Britain, BMJ, 3, 150-5.

Kohn, R. & White, K.L. (eds) 1976 Health-Care: An International Study, OUP, London.

Konotey-Ahulu, A. 1982 The Guardian, 8th January.

Koos, E. 1954 The Health of Regionville, Columbia Uni Press, New York.

Kosa, J.; Zola, I. & Antonovsky, A. 1969 Poverty and Health, Harvard, Mass.

Kotarba, J. 1983 Perceptions of death, Soc. Sci. & Med., 17, 10, 681-9.

Kroeber, P. & Kluckholm, C. 1968 in Singer, M. (ed) in International Encyclopaedia of Social Sciences, Macmillan, New York.

Lawrence, E. 1982a in CCCS, op.cit., 47-94.

Lawrence, E. 1982b in CCCS, op.cit., 95-142.

Learmonth, A. 1979 Factors in child burn and scald accidents, J. Epid. & Community Hlth, 33, 270-3.

Lee, T.R. 1977 Race and Residence, OUP, Oxford.

Lehmann, R 1974 Treatment of sickle-cell anaemia, BMJ, 2, A, 236-8.

Lerner, G. (ed) 1972 Black Women in White America, Pantheon Books, New York.

Lewis, D. 1973 Anthropology and Colonialism, Current Anthropology, 14,5, 581-592.

Lewis, G. 1981 in Eisenberg & Kleinman, op.cit., 151-162.

Littlewood, R & Cross, S 1980 Ethnic minorities and psychiatric services, Sociol. of Hlth & Illness, 2, 2, 194-201.

Littlewood, R & Lipsedge, M 1982 Aliens and Alienists, Penguin, Harmondsworth.

Livingstone, D. N. 1984 Nathaniel S. Shaler, Trans. IBG, NS 9, 2, 181-210.

Locker, D. 1981 Symptoms and Illness, Tavistock, London.

Louch, A.R. 1966 Explanation and Human Action, Uni. of California Press, L.A.

Lumb, K.M. et al | 1981 | Perinatal mortality, J. Epid. & Community Hlth., 35, 106-9.

Maccormack, C. | 1980 | Health care of ethnic minority groups, MIMS Magazine, 15th July, 53-60.

Manning, P.K. | 1967 | Problems in interpreting interview data, Sociology and Social Research, 51, 3, 302-16.

Mason, P. | 1970a | Patterns of Dominance, IRR, OUP, London.

Mason, P. | 1970b | Race Relations, OUP, London.

Maykovitch, M.K. | 1980 | Medical Sociology, Alfred, California.

Mays, N. | 1981 | Health needs of elderly Asians, Geriatric Med., 11, 11, 37-41.

McKeown, T. | 1976 | The Role of Medicine, Nuffield Provincial Trust, London.

McKinlay, J.B. | 1981 | in Eisenberg & Kleinman, op.cit., 77-107.

McKinney, J.C. & Tiryakian, E.A. (eds) | 1970 | Theoretical Sociology, Appleton-Century Crofts, New York.

Mechanic, D. | 1963 | Religion, religiosity and illness behaviour among Jews, Human Organisation, 22, 3, 202-6.

Mechanic, D. | 1978 | Medical Sociology, Free Press, New York.

Mennel, S. | 1974 | Sociological Theory - Uses and Unities, Nelson, London.

MIND | 1976 | Prevalence of Psychiatric Problems among Ethnic Minorities, MIND, London.

Mitchell, B. & Draper, D. | 1982 | Relevance and ethics in Geography, Longman, Essex.

Mitchell, J.C. | 1969 | Social Networks in Urban Situations, Manchester Uni Press, Manchester.

Mitchell, J.C. | 1983 | Case and Situational Analysis, Sociological Review, 31, 2, 187-211.

Modele, B. et al | 1980 | Introducing ante-natal diagnosis, BMJ, 280, 1347-50.

Moore, R. | 1975 | Racism and Black Resistance, Pluto Press, London.

Mueller, C. | 1970 | The repression of communicative behaviour, in Dreitzel, op.cit., 101-113.

Nader, L. & Maretzki, T. (eds) | 1973 | Cultural Illness and Health, Am. Anthropological Association, New York.

Nathan, P. & Leichleitner-Japanangka	1983	Health Business, Heinemann, Australia.
Navarro, V.	1978	Class Struggle, the State and Medicine, Martin Robertson, London.
Nichter, M.	1981	Idioms of distress, Culture, Medicine and Psychiatry, 5, 379-408.
OPCS	1982a	Population Trends, 28, Summer, HMSO.
OPCS	1982b	OPCS Monitor, LFS, 82, 1.
Oppe, T	1964	Medical problems of immigrant children, Proc. Royal Soc. Med., 57, 321-3.
Oppenheim, A.N.	1966	Questionnaire Design and attitude Measurement, Heinemann, London.
	1964	Oxford English Dictionary.
Paine, L.H. (ed)	1978	Health Care in Big Cities, Croom Helm, London.
Parkhouse, J.	1979	Medical Manpower in Britain, Churchill, Edinburgh.
Parkin, F.	1982	Max Weber, Tavistock, London.
Parmar, P.	1982	in CCCS, op.cit., 236-275.
Parry, W.H.	1970	Health and welfare of immigrants, Proc. Royal Soc. of Med., 63, 629-36.
Parsons, T.	1951	The Social System, Routledge and Kegan Paul, London.
Patterson, S.	1963	Immigrants in London, NCSS, London.
Patterson, S.	1964	Immigrants in London, Proc. Royal Soc. of Med., 57, 24-29.
Paul, B.D.	1955	Health, Culture and Community, Russel Sage, New York.
Peach, G.K.C.	1968	West Indian Migration to Britain, OUP, London.
Pearson, M	1983	The politics of ethnic minority health studies, Radical Community Med., Winter, 45-52.
Pedoe, H. et al	1975	Coronary heart attacks in East London, The Lancet, 2, ii, 833-8.
	1965	Penguin English Dictionary.
Pfifferling, J-H.	1981	in Eisenberg & Kleinman, op.cit., 197-222.
Phillips, D.L.	1973	Abandoning Method, Jossey-Bass, London.

Phillips, D.R. 1981 Contemporary Issues in the Geography of Health Care, Geo Books, Norwich.

Phillipson, M. 1972a Theory, methodology and conceptualisation, in Filmer, op.cit., 78-116.

Phillipson, M. 1972b Phenomenological philosophy and sociology, in Filmer, op.cit., 119-163.

Philpott, S.B. 1973 West Indian Migration: The Montserrat Case, Athlone Press, London.

Phizacklea, A. & Miles, R. 1980 Labour and Racism, Routledge and Kegan Paul, London.

Pietrek, S et al 1976 Prevention of vitamin D deficiency, The Lancet, 1, ii, 1145-8.

Pilisuk, M. & Froland, C. 1978 Social networks and illness, Soc. Sci. & Med., 12B, 273-8.

Pill, R. & Stott, N. 1982 Concepts of illness causation and responsibility, Soc. Sci. & Med., 16, 43-52.

Pillary, H.M. 1984 The concepts "causation", "racism" and "mental illness", Internat. J. of Soc. Psychology, 30, 1, 29-40.

Pless, I & Hood, C 1967 West Indian one year olds, The Lancet, June 24th, 1373-6.

Pocock, D.F. 1971 Social Anthropology, Sheed & Ward, London.

Pocock, D. 1975 Understanding Social Anthropology, Hodder and Stoughton, London.

Preece, M. et al 1973 Vitamin D deficiency, The Lancet, 1, 2, 907-10.

Pryce, K. 1979 Endless Pressure, Penguin, Harmondsworth.

Qureshi, B.A. 1981 Nutrition in multi-ethnic groups, Royal Society of Hlth J., 101, 5, 187-95.

Rack, P 1979 in Khan, V S Minority Families in Britain, Macmillan, London, 165-180

Rainwater, L. & Yancy, W. 1967 The Moynihan Report, MIT, Cambridge.

Rathwell, T. 1981 Health planning sensitive to ethnic minorities, Radical Community Medicine, 6, 3-6.

Rees, T. 1982 in Husband, op.cit., 75-96.

Rex, J. | 1983 | Race Relations in Sociological Theory, Routledge and Kegan Paul, London.

Rex, J. & Moore, R. | 1967 | Race, Community and Conflict, OUP, London.

Rex, J. & Tomlinson, S. | 1979 | Colonial Immigrants in a British City, Routledge and Kegan Paul, London.

Roberts, H. (ed) | 1981 | Doing Feminist Research, Routledge and Kegan Paul, London.

Robinson, D. | 1971 | The Process of Becoming Ill, Routledge & Kegan Paul, London.

Robinson, D. | 1973 | Patients, Practitioners and Medical Care, Heinemann, London.

Robinson, W.S. | 1951 | The logical structure of analytic induction, Am. Sociological Review, 16, 812-818.

Rodney, W. | 1972 | How Europe Underdeveloped Africa, Bogle L'Ouverture, London.

Rose, A.M. (ed) | 1962 | Human behaviour and social processes, Routledge and Kegan Paul, London.

Rose, E.J.B. (ed) | 1969 | Colour and Citizenship, OUP, London.

Rosenstock, I. | 1966 | in Millbank Memorial Fund Quarterly, 44, 94.

Runnymede Trust & Radical Statistics Race Group | 1980 | Britain's Black Population, Heinemann Educational Books, London.

Rushdie, S. | 1982 | The new empire within Britain, New Society, 62, 1047, 417-421.

Sarjeant, P | 1974 | Sickle-cell disease, BMJ, 2, A.

Sashidharan, S | 1981 | Unpub. paper, Symposium on ethnic minorities health, Imperial coll.

Saunders, L. | 1954 | Cultural Differences and Medical Care, Russel Sage, New York.

Schneider, D.M. | 1955 | in Paul, op.cit., 211-235.

Schofield, J | 1981 | Behind the veil, Health Visitor, 54, in three parts: 4,5 & 6; 138-41, 183-6, 248-51.

Schutz, A. | 1972 | The Phenomenology of the Social World, Heinemann Educational Books, London.

Schwartz, H. & Jacobs, J. | 1979 | Qualitative Sociology, Free Press, New York.

Shannon, G. & Dever, G.	1974	Health Care Delivery, McGraw Hill, New York.
Sheiham, H & Quick, A	1982	The Rickets Report, Haringey CHC & CRC, London.
Shyllon, F.D.	1977	Black People in Britain, 1555 - 1837, IRR, OUP, London.
Sickle Cell Society	1981	Sickle Cell Disease: The Need For Improved Services, Sickle Cell Society, London.
Sills, D. (ed)	1968	International Encyclopaedia of the Social Sciences, 11, 232-238, Macmillan, London.
Silverman, D.	1972a	Analysis of traditional sociology, in Filmer, op.cit, 1-12.
Silverman, D.	1972b	Some neglected questions about social reality, in Filmer, op.cit., 165-81.
Silverman, D.	1972c	Methodology and meaning, in Filmer, op.cit., 183-200.
Simon, R.	1982	Gramsci's Political Thought, Lawrence & Wishart, London.
Sivanandan, A.	1982	A Different Hunger, Pluto Press, London.
Sivanandan, A.	1983	Challenging Racism, Race and Class, XXV, 2, 1-11.
Skone, J.F.	1968	Public Health Aspects of Immigration, National Council for Civil Liberties.
Smith, A	1968	The Science of Social Medicine, Staple, London
Smith, D.J.	1977	Racial Disadvantage in Britain: The PEP Report, Penguin, Harmondsworth.
Smith, D.J.	1980	Overseas Doctors in the NHS, PSI, London.
Smith, D.M.	1977	Human Geography : A Welfare Approach, Edward Arnold, London.
Smith, D.M.	1979	Where the Grass is Greener, Penguin, Harmondsworth.
Snow, L.F.	1978	Black folk healers in urban America, Culture, Medicine and Psychiatry, 2, 69-106.
Spare Rib	1982	Caribbean Women, Spare Rib, October, 123.
Springett, V. et al	1958	TB in immigrants, Br.J.Prev.Soc.Med., 12, 135-40.

Springett, VH et al 1964 Tb in immigrants, The Lancet, 6th May, 1091-5.

Stacey, M. (ed) 1976 The Sociology of the NHS, Croom Helm.

Stanley, N.F. & Joske, R.A. (eds) 1980 Changing Disease patterns and Human Behaviour, Academic Press, London.

Stephens, W. et al 1981 High dose vitamin D, The Lancet, 2, 8257, 1199-1201.

Stimson, G.V. & Webb, B. 1975 Going to See the Doctor, Routledge and Kegan Paul, London.

Stoeckle, J.D. & Barsky, A.J. 1981 in Eisenberg & Kleinman, op.cit, 223-40.

Stopes-Roe, M. & Cochrane, R. 1980 Mental health and integration, Ethnic and Racial Studies, 3, 3, 316-41.

Suchman, E.A. 1964 Socio-medical variations among ethnic groups, Am. J. of Sociology, 70, 319-31.

Sudnow, D. 1967 Passing On, Prentice Hall, New Jersey.

Susser, M.W. & Watson, W. 1971 Sociology in Medicine, OUP, London.

Swan, C.& Cooke, W. 1971 Nutritional osteomalacia, The Lancet, 2, i, 456-8.

Szymanski, A. 1971 Toward a radical sociology, in Colfax and Roach, op.cit 93-107.

Tabor, D.C. 1981 Ripe and unripe, Soc. Sci. and Med., 15B, 439-55.

Terry, P. et al 1980 Ethnic differences in perinatal stats, BMJ, 281, 1307-8.

Thalassaemia Society 1981 Stamp Out Thalassaemia, Thalassaemia Society, London.

Thomas, HE 1968 TB in Britain, Proc. Royal Soc.Med., 61.

Times 1981 Sickle cell disease detectable in embryo, The Times, 17th October.

Torkington, P. 1983 The Racial Politics of Health, Uni Liverpool.

Totman, R. 1979 Social Causes of Ill-Health, Souvenir, London.

Townsend, P. 1979 Poverty in the UK, Penguin, Harmondsworth.

Townsend, P. & Davidson, N. 1982 Inequalities in Health, Penguin, Harmondsworth.

Tremblay, M-A. 1982 The key informant, in Burgess, op.cit., 98-104.

Turner, V.W. 1957 A Study of Ndembu Village Life, Manchester University Press, Manchester.

Twaddle, A.C. 1981 in Eisenberg & Kleinman, op.cit., 111-133.

Twaddle, A.C. & Hessler, R.M. 1977 A Sociology of Health, CV Moseby, St. Louis.

Urry, J. 1981 The Anatomy of Capitalist Societies, Macmillan, London.

Van-Velsen, J. 1967 The extended case method, in Epstein, A.L. (ed) The Craft of Social Anthropology, Tavistock, London.

Wadsworth, MEJ, et al 1971 Health and Sickness: The Choice of Treatment, Tavistock, London.

Walsh, D. 1972a Sociology in the social world, in Filmer, op.cit., 15-35.

Walsh, D. 1972b Varieties of positivism, in Filmer, op.cit., 37-55.

Walsh, D. 1972c Functionalism and systems theory, in Filmer, op.cit., 57-74.

Walters, V. 1980 Class Inequality and Health Care, Croom Helm, London.

Watson, J.L. (ed) 1977 Between Two Cultures, Blackwell, Oxford.

Waxler, N.E. 1977 Mental illness in traditional societies, Culture, Medicine and Psychiatry, 1, 233-53.

Webb, P 1981 Health problems of London's Asians and Afro-Caribbeans, Health Visitor, 54, 4, 141-7.

Whyte, W.F. 1982 Interviewing, in Burgess, op.cit., 111-122.

Widgery, D. 1979 Health in Danger, Macmillan, London.

Williams, R. 1958 Cuture and Society, Penguin, Harmondsworth.

Wilson, A. 1978 Finding a Voice, Virago, London.

Wilson, A. 1981 NHS may rule out blacks, New Statesman, 101, 13-14.

Wilson, M. 1951 Witch beliefs and social structure, Am. J. of Sociology, 45.

Wilson, W.J. 1973 Power, Race and Privilege, Macmillan, New York.

Winch, P. 1958 The Idea of a Social Science, Routledge and Kegan Paul, London.

Wolstenholme, C. & O'Connor, M. (eds) 1966 Immigrants : Medical and Social Aspects, Ciba Foundation Report, Churchill, London.

Wright, C. 1981 Maternal and child health, 6, 427-30.

Wright, D.R. 1983 Contemp. Issues in Geog. and Educ., 1, 1, 12-15.

Young, M. et al 1981 Report from Hackney, PSI, London.

Yudkin, S. 1968 Health and Welfare of the immigrant child, National Council for Civil Liberties.

Zborowski, M. 1952 Cultural components in responses to pain, J. of Social Issues, 8, 16-30.

Zola, I.K. 1966 Culture and symptoms, Am. Sociological Review, 31, 615-30.

Zola, I.K. 1975a in Cox & Mead, op.cit., 23-48.

Zola, I.K. 1975b in Cox & Mead, op.cit., 170-185.

Zola, I.K. 1981 in Eisenberg & Kleinman, op.cit., 241-252.

Zubaida, S. (ed) 1970 Race and Racialism, Tavistock, London.